THE NEW CORGI
CALORIE COUNTER

THE NEW CORGI

CALORIE

COUNTER

ANNE BEWLEY

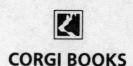

CORGI BOOKS

THE NEW CORGI CALORIE COUNTER
A CORGI BOOK 0 552 14203 4

First publication in Great Britain

PRINTING HISTORY
Corgi edition published 1989
Corgi edition reprinted 1989
Corgi edition reprinted 1991
Corgi edition reprinted 1992
Corgi edition (revised and updated) reissued 1994

Set in Monotype Gill by Phoenix Typesetting, Ilkley

Corgi Books are published by Transworld Publishers Ltd,
61–63 Uxbridge Road, Ealing, London W5 5SA,
in Australia by Transworld Publishers (Australia) Pty Ltd,
15–25 Helles Avenue, Moorebank, NSW 2170,
and in New Zealand by Transworld Publishers (NZ) Ltd,
3 William Pickering Drive, Albany, Auckland.

Printed and bound in Great Britain by
Cox & Wyman Ltd, Reading, Berks.

CONTENTS

DRINK

ACKNOWLEDGEMENTS

Many of the calorific values in this book are taken from *The Composition of Foods* by R. A. McCance and E. M. Widdowson, fourth revised and extended edition of the Medical Research Council Special Report No 297 by A. A. Paul and D. A. T. Southgate published by HMSO, Crown copyright 1978, third impression 1985.

The author would like to thank Susan Collins for all her help with the project, together with Clare Whittaker, Wendy Beveridge and Elaine Koster.

INTRODUCTION

One of the most popular ways to control weight is to limit the number of calories that you take in each day. Counting is not difficult and the results from a calorie-controlled diet are often more satisfactory than those achieved on one of the crash diets. Despite the ever-growing number of meal replacement foods that come on to the market, many people return to the simple method of counting the calories each day in the foods that they eat to achieve success in weight control. This book is for them.

A calorie is simply a unit of energy. The body requires a certain number each day to function. Using up the same number of units a day as you consume in food means that your weight should remain constant. To lose weight, the balance has to be tipped. Each of us has a different metabolic rate. Someone doing a job which requires a considerable amount of physical labour will burn up more units of energy than someone who sits at an office desk all day. For a woman the average number of calories used up in a day varies from 2,250 to 1,750. For a man, the number varies from 3,500 to 2,500. When first going on to a calorie-controlled diet it is sensible to aim at eating foods that contain 250 calories

less than the average for a couple of weeks; if you lose
1–2 kg (2–3½ lb) in the first week and slightly less in the
second week, that should be satisfactory. It is probable that
you will lose extra fluid from the body during the first week,
which explains why the weight loss is greater. By eating 250
calories fewer than you use up, it is probable that you will
break down approximately 25 g (1 oz) of solid fat from the
body's stores.

If at the end of two weeks you have not lost weight, then
the number of calories you take in each day should be cut
slightly more, say by 400 units a day.

Tips for weight loss

*Try to eat your main meal in the middle of the day. This
gives you the rest of the day in which to expend energy and
use up the calories you have consumed. Fewer calories are
used up when you are asleep.

*Eat food slowly. This has the effect of making you feel more
satisfied than if you gobble food in a rush.

*Keep a weekly chart of your progress. This is encouraging
and should help to stop you breaking your diet. Do not rush
to the scales every day as this can be disappointing.

*Keep to a healthy diet, a well-balanced mixture of protein,
carbohydrate and fats. It is wise to cut down on carbo-
hydrates and fatty foods as these tend to contain more
calories but do not exclude them altogether, as they are
essential in some measure to good health.

*Never nibble in between meals, and try to make yourself as varied a diet as possible; this can help you to avoid temptation.

*Do not worry if you exceed your allowance of calories one day; you can compensate for it the next day by reducing your intake by the total over-consumed. But do not allow this to happen frequently. Be honest with yourself.

*Weight loss occurs when you eat less. In other words, to lose weight you need to reduce your intake of calories.

I hope that you find this book helps you.

NOTE

The products in this book have been arranged into groups such as Biscuits, Bread, Burgers, Confectionery, Diabetic, Meat, Simply for Slimmers, Soups, Vegetarian in the Food Section and Beer & Lager, Crushes, Hot Drinks, Slimmers' and Health Drinks, Wines in the Drink Section.

Where a product is made by several manufacturers I have included a range of them, particularly those where the calorific content varies from one manufacturer to another. I should like to thank all the manufacturers who have kindly helped by providing calorie counts for this book.

WHAT YOU SHOULD WEIGH

This is a mean average of what you should weigh and may be helpful in giving you a target to work to. Large or small-framed people can add or deduct weight from these figures, but be sure you do not cheat.

WOMEN

4ft 10in	1.47m	7st 3lb	45.5 kg
4ft 11in	1.50m	7st 6lb	47.0 kg
5ft	1.52m	7st 9lb	48.5 kg
5ft 1in	1.55m	7st 12lb	50.0 kg
5ft 2in	1.57m	8st 1lb	51.0 kg
5ft 3in	1.60m	8st 4lb	52.5 kg
5ft 4in	1.63m	8st 7lb	54.0 kg
5ft 5in	1.65m	8st 11lb	55.75kg
5ft 6in	1.68m	9st 1lb	57.5 kg
5ft 7in	1.70m	9st 5lb	59.25kg
5ft 8in	1.73m	9st 9lb	61.0 kg
5ft 9in	1.75m	9st 13lb	63.0 kg
5ft 10in	1.78m	10st 3lb	64.5 kg
5ft 11in	1.80m	10st 7lb	66.5 kg
6ft	1.83m	10st 11lb	68.5 kg

WHAT YOU SHOULD WEIGH

MEN

5ft 2in	1.57m	8st 11lb	55.5kg
5ft 3in	1.60m	9st 1lb	57.5kg
5ft 4in	1.63m	9st 4lb	59.0kg
5ft 5in	1.65m	9st 7lb	60.0kg
5ft 6in	1.68m	9st 10lb	61.5kg
5ft 7in	1.70m	10st	63.5kg
5ft 8in	1.73m	10st 5lb	65.5kg
5ft 9in	1.75m	10st 9lb	67.5kg
5ft 10in	1.78m	10st 13lb	69.5kg
5ft 11in	1.80m	11st 3lb	71.0kg
6ft	1.83m	11st 8lb	73.5kg
6ft 1in	1.85m	11st 12lb	75.0kg
6ft 2in	1.88m	12st 3lb	77.5kg
6ft 3in	1.90m	12st 8lb	79.5kg
6ft 4in	1.93m	12st 13lb	82.0kg

FOOD

	g	oz	Cal.

BISCUITS, SAVOURY AND CRISPBREADS

Bran Crispbread, GG Scandinavian Suppliers	each		12
Bran or Sesame Thin Crispbread, Ideal	each		15
Brown Crispbread, Ryvita	each		25
Brown Crispbread, Ry-King	each		30
Butter Puff, Crawfords	each		52
Carr's Table Water Biscuit:			
large	each		30
small	each		16
Cheddar Savoury Biscuit, Crawfords	each		21
Cheeselets, Peak Frean	each		3
Cheese Ritz Crackers, Nabisco	each		15
Cheese Sandwich Biscuit, Waitrose	28	1	140
Cheese Snack Pack, Crawfords	each		154

		g	oz	Cal.
Cheese Thins, Gateway	each			21
Cracker Barrel Biscuit, Kraft		28	1	114
Cream Cracker Biscuit:				
Jacobs	each			33
Waitrose		28	1	122
Energen	slice			18
Fine Highland Triangle, Nairn's	each			76
High Baked Water Biscuit, Tesco	each			20
Krackawheat Biscuit, McVitie's	each			37
Macvita Crispbread, McVitie's	each			35
Savours Savoury Biscuit, Crawfords	packet	35	1¼	195
Scanda Crisps, GG Scandinavian Suppliers	slice			18
Sesame Cracker, Waitrose		28	1	138
Superfine Matzos, Rakusen's	each			74
Table Water Biscuit, Carr's:				
large	each			30
small	each			16
TUC	each			26

	g	oz	Cal.
TUC, Savoury Sandwich Biscuit, McVitie's	each		78
Water High Bake Biscuit, Jacobs	each		21
Wheat Crackers, Tesco	each		18
Whole Grain Crispbread, Ideal	each		10
Wholemeal Bran Biscuit, St Michael	each		60
Wholemeal Bran, Safeway	each		64
Wholemeal Thins, Sainsbury	each		12

BISCUITS, SWEET

	g	oz	Cal.
Abbey Crunch, McVitie's	each		47
Affairs, Chocolate, Huntley & Palmer	28	1	137
All Butter Shortbread Finger, St Michael	each		110
All Butter Crunch, Sainsbury	each		30
All Butter Thins, Safeway	each		19
Almond & Honey, McVitie's	each		86
Animals, Cadbury	each		30

FOOD

	g	oz	Cal.
Balmoral Shortbread, Crawfords	each		66
Bandit, McVitie's	each		103
Bargain Bag Choc Chip & Hazelnut Cookies, Crawfords	each		40
Big 5 Caramel Wafer, Spar	28	1	136
Bran, Allinson	each		53
Bourbon Cream: Peak Frean	each		56
Rakusen's	each		58
Bournville Digestive, Cadbury	each		45
Bran, Boots Second Nature	each		123
Bran Wholemeal, Fox's	each		64
Brandy Snap, St Michael	each		25
Butterlace, Huntley & Palmer	each		38
Butter Crunch Cream Biscuit, St Michael	each		143
Butterscotch Teamates, Paterson	each		60
Butter Shortcake, Fox's	each		82
Caramel Wafer, Tunnocks	each		125
Caramel Wafer, Mackintosh	each		85

BISCUITS 25

		g	oz	Cal.
Carob Chip, Prewetts	each			85
Cherry, Granose	each	45	1½	170
Choc 'n' Nut Cookie, Gateway	each			52
Chocolate Biscuit Finger, milk or plain, McVitie's	each			25
Chocolate Chip Cookie, Gateway	each			51
Chocolate Digestive, plain, St Michael	each			143
Chocolate Homewheat, milk or plain, McVitie's	each			84
Chocolate Orange Cookie, Waitrose	each			40
Citrus Fruit Crunch, Co-op	each			59
Coconut Cookie, Huntley & Palmer	each			80
Coconut Crumble Cream, Waitrose		28	1	146
Coconut Macaroon, Tesco	each			50
Coconut Mallow, Peak Frean	each			46
Coconut Rings, Tesco	each			45
Coffee Cream, Peak Frean	each			57

FOOD

	g	oz	Cal.
Cookie Coaster, Cadbury	each		45
Country Crunch, Peak Frean	each		36
Crunch Cream, Peak Frean	each		57
Crunchy Oat, Slimmers	each		63
Custard Cream: Tesco	each		66
Safeway	each		64
Devon Cream, Peak Frean	each		55
Digestive:			
Burtons	each		50
Bournville, Cadbury	each		45
Chocolate, Huntley & Palmer	each		60
Chocolate, Sainsbury	each		60
Fruit, Huntley & Palmer	each		50
Hovis	each		57
Huntley & Palmer	each		65
McVitie's	each		73
Milk chocolate: Cadbury	each		50
St Michael	each		65
Sainsbury	each		60
Plain chocolate: St Michael	each		65
Fig Roll, Jacobs	each		50
Garibaldi, Sainsbury	each		30
Ginger Crunch Cream, Fox's	each		68
Ginger Nut, McVitie's	each		45

	g	oz	Cal.
Ginger Snap, Sainsbury	each		40
Golden Crunch, Paterson	each		55
Granny Ann HiFi, Itona	each		125
Gipsy Cream, McVitie's	each		67
Happy Bear Honey, McVitie's	each		114
Healthy Life, Mitchelhill	each		61
Highland Finger, Crawfords	each		66
Hobnob, Milk Chocolate, McVitie's	each		80
Honey, Allinson	each		55
Iced Gem, Peak Frean	each		7
Iced Shorties, Crawfords Pennywise	each		40
Jaffa Cake: McVitie's	each		47
Sainsbury	each		45
Jaffa Crunch, Peak Frean	each		30
Jamboree Mallow, Peak Frean	each		75
Jam Sandwich Cream, Fox's	each		74
Jammie Dodger, Burton's	each		84
Jersey Cream, Peak Frean	each		55
Lemon Crisp, Tesco	each		42

	g	oz	Cal.
Lemon Crumble Cream, Spar	28	1	147
Lemon Marshmallows, Barker & Dobson	28	1	92
Lemon Puff, Sainsbury	each		75
Lincoln, McVitie's	each		42
Macdonalds Taxi, McVitie's	each		75
Malted Milk Chocolate Bar, Elkes	each		95
Marie, Crawfords	each		32
Milk Chocolate Finger, Safeway	each		45
Milk Chocolate Orange Finger, Safeway	each		48
Milk Chocolate Assorted, Cadbury	each		62
Milk Chocolate Tea Cake, St Michael	each		80
Morning Coffee, Tesco	each		21
Muesli, Allinson	each		62
Muesli Slice, Holly Mills	each		216
Munchmallow, McVitie's	each		79
Neapolitan Wafer, Peak Frean	each		32

		g	oz	Cal.
Nice Cream, Peak Frean	each			57
Oatcakes, average		28	1	125
Oat, Fruit & Nut, Holly Mills	each			174
Oatmeal: Allinson	each			60
Country Basket	each			35
Oatmeal Crunch, Sainsbury	each			35
Orange Club, Jacobs	each			115
Orange Cream:				
Cadbury	each			80
Peak Frean	each			55
Orange Milk Chocolate Waifa, Terry's	each			180
Orange Viscount, Burton's	each			90
Original Thick Tea, Fox's	each			62
Penguin, McVitie's	each			127
Petticoat Tail, Sainsbury	each			50
Picnic Bar, Cadbury	each			220
Plain Chocolate Wafer, Terry's	each			175
Plain Chocolate Ginger, St Michael	each			64
Rich Highland Shortie, Nisa	each			50

	g	oz	Cal.
Rich Tea: Burton's	each		36
Sainsbury	each		45
Rich Tea Finger, Sainsbury	each		25
Rich Tea Finger Cream, St Michael	each		50
Sesame and Sunflower, Prewetts	each		85
Shortbread Fingers, Littlewoods	each		95
Shortbread Round, Paterson	each		500
Shortcake: Presto	each		60
Safeway	each		70
Six Grain, Boots Second Nature, Wholemeal	each		40
Snapjack, Fruit, Burton's	each		72
Snowball: Burton's	each		105
Sainsbury	each		105
Sponge Finger, Huntley & Palmer	each		20
Sports, Fox's	each		32
Stem Ginger, Prewetts	each		78
Sprinters, Sainsbury	each		105
Sultana Cookie, St Michael	each		54

	g	oz	Cal.
Sultana and Date Cookie, Peak Frean	pack		75
Sunnybisk, Granose	each		70
Thick Finger Shortbread, Burton's	each		103
Thin Arrowroot, Crawfords	each		32
Thistle Shortbread, Burton's	each		105
Traditional Brandy Snap, Fox's	each		57
Traditional Malt Bake, McVitie's	each		35
Traditional Nice, Crawfords	each		25
Treacle Crunch Cream, Fox's	each		67
Trio, Jacob's	each		126
United Golden Crunch, McVitie's	each		102
United Orange, McVitie's	each		102
Wafer, Crawfords	each		40
Wafer Delight, Huntley & Palmer	each		97
Walnut/Orange Cookie, Waitrose	each		146
Wholemeal, Slimmers Healthy Life Range	each		74

		g	oz	Cal.
Wholemeal Shortbread, Boots Second Nature	each			100
Wholemeal Shortbread Finger, Waitrose		28	1	141
Yoghurt, Country Basket	each			34
Yo Yo, McVitie's: mint	each			99
toffee	each			95

BREAD

		g	oz	Cal.
Baguette		28	1	70
Big Country Bread, St Michael		28	1	66
Big T White, Mothers Pride	slice			115
Black rye		28	1	94
Brown		28	1	63
Currant		28	1	70
Fried in lard	slice	28	1	160
French	slice	28	1	85
French wholemeal		28	1	70
Fruit sesame		28	1	120
Granary	slice	28	1	70

		g	oz	Cal.
HiBran, Vitbe, small loaf	slice			55
High Fibre Wholemeal Loaf	slice			71
Laver		28	1	15
Malted Wheat Cob, Sainsbury		28	1	66
Malty Brown, Nimble	slice			50
Milk	slice			86
Nut Loaf, Granose		425	15	750
Pumpernickel	slice	28	1	64
Rye-Bran, Primula: extra thin	slice			15
thick	slice			19
Soda, white	slice			80
Sunmalt Loaf, Sunblest		28	1	74
Wheaten Brown Bread, Fine Lady	slice			78
Wheatgerm	slice			70
Wheatmeal Bread Mix, Granny Smith	pack			835
White		28	1	69
White Bread Mix, Granny Smith	pack			1000
Wholemeal, average		28	1	78

		g	oz	Cal.
Wholemeal, 100%	slice			66
Breadcrumbs: dried	15ml/1 tablespoon			30
fresh	15ml/1 tablespoon			8

BREAD ROLLS AND BUNS

		g	oz	Cal.
Bagel	each	40	1½	150
Bap	each	40	1½	135
Bath bun	each	40	1½	122
Breadstick	each			15
Bridge roll	each	15	½	35
Brioche	each	40	1½	196
Chelsea bun	each	90	3¼	250
Croissant	each	40	1½	165
Crumpet, toasted	each	40	1½	75
Currant bun	each	40	1½	137
French toast	slice			50
Hot cross bun	each	40	1½	160
Hovis roll	each	40	1½	100

		g	oz	Cal.
Muffin	each	60	2¼	125
Pitta	standard	70	2½	186
Roll, Starch Reduced, Energen	each			25
Scone, white	each	50	2	206
Teacake	each	50	2	152
Savoury bun, Daloon	pack			130

BURGERS

		g	oz	Cal.
American Hamburger, Brooks	each			315
Baconburger, Wimpy	each			302
Baked Beans with Hamburgers, Chef		28	1	34
Beefburger: average minus bun		28	1	55
Birds Eye, Original (Burger in a Bun)	pack			335
100%	each			120
Iceland, 100%, with bun, grilled	each			119
Waitrose, frozen		28	1	90
Big Mac with Bun, McDonald's	each			446

	g	oz	Cal.
Burger, Birds Eye Economy each			100
Cheeseburger with Bun, McDonald's each			272
Cheeseburger with Bun, Wimpy each			305
Egg and Bacon in a Bun, Wimpy each			430
Fish Burgers, Birds Eye each			95
Hamburger:			
Danish Prime each			120
in gravy, Tesco tinned	28	1	36
Waitrose each, frozen			146
with Bun, McDonald's each			223
Minceburger, cooked without fat, Birds Eye each			100
Quarter Pounder with Bun, McDonald's each			400
Quarter Pounder with Cheese & Bun, McDonald's each			492
Rather Special Beefburgers, McLaren each			204
Turkey & Beefburger, Matthew's, grilled with no fat each			270

	g	oz	Cal.
Wimpy Kingsize, Wimpy	each		405
Wimpy Half-pounder in bun, Wimpy	each		830
Wimpy Quarter-pounder with bun, Wimpy	each		530
Wimpy Quarter-pounder with bun & cheese, Wimpy	each		575

CAKES AND SCONES

	g	oz	Cal.
All Butter Eccles Cake, Waitrose	28	1	118
All Butter Walnut Sandwich Cake, Sainsbury, large	28	1	115
Angel Layer Cake, Mr Kipling	28	1	101
Apple & Blackcurrant 6 Fruit Pie, Lyons	each		376
Apricot & Cream Macaroons, St Michael	each		439
Bakewell Slice, Mr Kipling, small cake	each		162
Battenburg, Lyons, large	each		990
Bavarian Cake, Green's	cake		1590

		g	oz	Cal.
Bisquick, Betty Crocker mix	packet			4800
Black Forest Gâteau:				
McVitie's		28	1	76
Tesco		28	1	87
Buttercream Walnut Cake, Mr Kipling		28		112
Butterfly Tops, Mary Baker Simply Sweet mix, Nabisco Frear	pack			840
Butter Madeira Cake, Lyons	each			337
Butter Cherry Genoa Cake, Safeway		28	1	94
Carnival, Viota cake mix, made up		28	1	110
Carrot Cake, Waitrose		28	1	108
Cherry Bakewell, Mr Kipling small cake	each			202
Cherry Genoa Cut, Safeway		28	1	90
Cherry Shortcake, Mary Baker mix, Nabisco Frear	packet			1383
Cherry Slice, Mr Kipling	each			129
Chocolate Cake, Cadbury		28	1	108
Chocolate Fudge Cake, Lyons	each			423

	g	oz	Cal.
Chocolate Continental Sponge Roll, Lyons	28	1	104
Chocolate Sponge Sandwich Cake, Tesco	each		1022
Coconut Macaroon, Mr Kipling small cake	each		116
Coffee Gâteau, Cadbury large cake	28	1	108
Congratulations Cake, St Michael	28	1	90
Cup Cake, Lyons: chocolate	each		129
orange & cream	each		129
Currant cake, average	28	1	119
Cut Cherry Genoa Cake, Safeway	28	1	90
Cut Sultana Cake, Safeway	28	1	101
Dark Chocolate Fudge Creamy Frostings Cake, Betty Crocker mix	28	1	90
Date & Walnut Wholemeal Cake mix, Granose			45
Devil's Food Cake, Betty Crocker mix	28	1	92

	g	oz	Cal.
Devon Sponge Cake, Green's mix	28	1	103
Doughnut, Sunblest	each		260
Dundee Cake, Waitrose	28	1	100
Eccles Cake: Mothers Pride	each		288
Sainsbury	28	1	112
Farmhouse Cake, Asda	28	1	110
Flake Cake, Cadbury	each		132
Flapjacks, Sainsbury	each		120
Fondant Fancy, Sainsbury small cake	each		106
French Fancy, Mr Kipling small cake	each		102
Fruit Loaf: Green's mix	packet		1390
Mary Baker Simply Sweet mix	packet		1190
Fruity Malt Loaf, Sainsbury	28	1	73
Fudge Brownie Mix, Betty Crocker mix	packet		2400
Chocolate Fudge Slice, Mr Kipling	each		135
Ginger Cake: Safeway	28	1	90
Viota mix	packet		975

	g	oz	Cal.
Gingerbread, average	28	1	105
Golden Cake, Betty Crocker mix	28	1	90
Golden Shred Orange Marmalade Cake, Viota mix	packet		1120
Harlequins, Mr Kipling	each		146
Honey Cake, Waitrose	28	1	120
Iced Bavarian Cake, Green's luxury mix	packet		2125
Iced Fairy Cakes, Viota mix	packet		1040
	each		108
Iced Fruit Cake, Sainsbury, large	28	1	94
Iced Madeira Sandwich Cake, Waitrose, large	28	1	121
Iced Rich Fruit Cake, Tesco	each		2027
Jaffa Finger, Mr Kipling small cake	each		133
Jam Doughnuts, Windmill	each		225
Jamaica Ginger Cake, Lyons large	each		1030
Jam Swiss Roll, Mr Kipling	28		59

	g	oz	Cal.
Junior Choc Roll, Cadbury:			
with caramel filling	each		125
with raspberry filling	each		114
Junior Jam Roll, Sainsbury	each		90
Lancashire Eccles Cake, Sainsbury	each		147
Lemon Cake Mix, Betty Crocker mix	packet		3120
Lemon Cup Cakes with water icing, Viota mix	packet		995
Lemon Madeira Cake, Granny Smith mix	each		915
Lemon Tops, Nabisco mix	each		830
Luxury Sponge Cake, Granny Smith mix	packet		1000
Madeira Cake: Green's mix	packet		1477
Mr Kipling	28	1	91
Manor House Cake, Mr Kipling	28	1	152
Marble Cake, Asda	28	1	102
Marzipan Top Christmas Cake, McVitie's	28	1	78

	g	oz	Cal.
Meringue Cream Cake, St Michael	28	1	99
Milk Chocolate Birthday Cake, St Michael	28	1	118
Milk Chocolate Cake, Betty Crocker mix	packet		2030
Milk Chocolate Roll, Waitrose	28	1	133
Mince Pies, Mr Kipling	each		207
Mini Jam Roll, Cadbury	28	1	114
Orange cake, plain, average	28	1	132
Orange Curl, Sainsbury	each		135
Orange Frosted Cake, Viota mix, made up	packet		1060
Orange Tops, Mary Baker mix	packet		831
Paradise Cake, Waitrose	28	1	29
Paradise Slice, Lyons	28	1	136
Plain Sponge Cake, Green's mix	packet		748
Profiteroles with sauce, Birds Eye	each		70
Queen's cake, average	28	1	129
Raspberry Sponge, Safeway	each		103

	g	oz	Cal.
Real Chocolate Fancy, Mr Kipling	each			92
Red Cherry Butter Sponge Cake, Tiffany's	each			300
Rice Crisp Cake with Raisins, St Michael	each			90
Rich Chocolate Madeira Sandwich, Sainsbury	each			1080
Rock Cake: Homepride	each			103
Tesco cake mix		28	1	99
Scone:				
Granny Smith mix	packet			865
Whitworth's mix		28	1	35
Snowball, St Michael	each			105
Sour Cream Chocolate Fudge Cake, Betty Crocker mix	packet			2040
Spicy Mix Cake, Granny Smith	packet			960
Stollen with Marzipan, Waitrose		28	1	107
Swiss Gâteau, Cadbury		28	1	112
Swiss Roll:				
black cherry & buttercream, Sainsbury, large	each			840
chocolate, Cadbury		28	1	113

	g	oz	Cal.
chocolate, Lyons each			630
raspberry, Sainsbury	28	1	83
raspberry & vanilla, Lyons each			625
Teacakes, Tesco mix packet			1320
Trifle Sponge Sandwich Cake, Lyons each			80
Trifle Sponge, Sainsbury	28	1	86
Vanilla Sandwich Cake, Mary Baker mix packet			1370
Victoria Sponge Cake:			
Homepride	28	1	127
Cadbury	28	1	64
Viennese Cake, St Michael each			283
Viennese Whirls, Lyons	28	1	143
Walnut Layer Cake:			
Viota mix, large packet			1247
Waitrose	28	1	115
White Chocolate Torte, St Michael	28	1	106

		g	oz	Cal.

CAKE DECORATIONS AND BAKING INGREDIENTS

		g	oz	Cal.
Angelica		28	1	90
Chocolate vermicelli		28	1	135
Coconut, desiccated		28	1	171
Crunch Base, Granny Smith mix		28	1	135
Baking powder	1 teaspoon			5
		28	1	45
Flour:				
brown		28	1	90
buckwheat		28	1	100
cornmeal, 96%		28	1	103
60%		28	1	100
cassava		28	1	97
granary		28	1	99
maizemeal, 96%		28	1	103
60%		28	1	100
rice		28	1	100
rye		28	1	95
soya: full fat		28	1	127
low fat		28	1	100
wheatmeal		28	1	93
white: plain		28	1	99
self-raising		28	1	96
strong		28	1	96

		g	oz	Cal.
wholemeal		28	1	90
yam		28	1	90
Hundreds & thousands, average	1 teaspoon			15
Jelly Crystals, Pearce Duff	packet			180
Jelly Diamonds, Pearce Duff		28	1	80
Kake Drops, Kakebrand		28	1	155
Marzipan, average		28	1	125
Polka Dots, Lyons Tetley: milk	packet			575
plain	packet			585
Simply Topping, Royal	packet			485
Sugar Flowers, Pearce Duff		28	1	105
Vanilla Top 'n' Fill, Homepride	sachet	220	7¾	940
Yeast: dried		28	1	48
fresh		28	1	15

CEREALS

		g	oz	Cal.
All-Bran, Kellogg's		28	1	78
Alpen, Weetabix		28	1	105
Alpen with Tropical Fruit, Weetabix		28	1	109

	g	oz	Cal.
Apple & Banana Bran Breakfast, Holly Mills	28	1	125
Apricot Wheats, Sainsbury	28	1	150
Barley, pearl, average: boiled	28	1	34
raw 1 tablespoon			45
Bran, average	28	1	58
Bran Buds, Kellogg's	28	1	78
Bran Fare, Weetabix	28	1	71
Bran Flakes, Co-op	28	1	98
Bran Muesli, Prewetts	28	1	90
Breakfast Oats, Prewetts	28	1	104
Breakfast Special, St Michael	28	1	107
Buckwheat	28	1	28
Crispy Muesli, Jordans	28	1	70
Cornflakes, Kellogg's	28	1	104
Coco Pops, Kellogg's	28	1	106
Crunchy Bran with Malt and Honey, Allinson	28	1	104
Crunchy Nut Cornflakes, Kellogg's	28	1	109

	g	oz	Cal.
Crunchy Oat & Cinnamon Flake, St Michael	28	1	120
Deluxe Muesli, Sunwheel Foods	28	1	110
Force Wheat Flakes	28	1	105
Flour:			
brown	28	1	90
buckwheat	28	1	100
cornmeal, 96%	28	1	103
60%	28	1	100
cassava	28	1	97
granary	28	1	99
maizemeal, 96%	28	1	103
60%	28	1	100
rice	28	1	100
rye	28	1	95
soya: full fat	28	1	127
low fat	28	1	100
wheatmeal	28	1	93
white: plain	28	1	99
self-raising	28	1	96
strong	28	1	96
wholemeal	28	1	90
yam	28	1	90
Frosties, Kellogg's	28	1	106
Ghosts & Bats, St Michael	28	1	101
Golden Crunch Breakfast, Mapleton's	28	1	124

	g	oz	Cal.
Golden Oatmeal Crisp, Kellogg's	28	1	108
Grape Nuts, Bird's	28	1	97
Harvest Break, Nabisco Frear	portion		220
Harvest Crunch, Tropical, Quaker	28	1	134
Honey Nut Loops, Kellogg's	28	1	107
Hot Bran, Quaker	28	1	92
Hot Oat with Bran, Sainsbury	28	1	103
Instant Hot Oat Cereal, Sainsbury	28	1	103
Tesco, without milk or sugar	28	1	118
Instant Porridge, Waitrose	28	1	115
Jumblies, Tesco	28	1	114
Maize	28	1	103
Muesli: average	28	1	106
Boots	28	1	98
Holly Mill, Sugar free	28	1	101
St Michael, Luxury	28	1	97
Oat & Apple Bran, Asda	28	1	90
Oatmeal: average, raw	28	1	114
Whitworth's	28	1	115

	g	oz	Cal.
Organic Grade Porridge Oats, Jordans	28	1	124
Porridge Oats:			
Co-op	28	1	102
Nisa	28	1	110
Whitworth's, uncooked	28	1	112
Puffed Rice, Tesco	28	1	106
Puffed Wheat: Quaker	28	1	92
Sainsbury	28	1	88
Quaker Oats, Quaker	28	1	105
Raisin Splitz, Kellogg's	28	1	90
Rice, brown: boiled	28	1	30
raw	28	1	100
white: boiled	28	1	35
raw	28	1	102
Rice Crunchies, Safeway	28	1	102
Rice Krispies, Kellogg's	28	1	106
Ricicles, Kellogg's	28	1	106
Sago, average, raw	28	1	102
Scotch Porridge Oats:			
Sainsbury	28	1	94
Tesco	28	1	108
Semolina, average, raw	28	1	99

	g	oz	Cal.
Special K, Kellogg's	28	1	104
Sugar Puffs, Quaker	28	1	104
Sultana Bran, Kellogg's	28	1	87
Summer Orchard, Kellogg's	28	1	123
Sunny Grains, Mapleton's	28	1	130
Swiss Style Breakfast:			
Safeway	28	1	116
Sainsbury	28	1	96
Tapioca, average, dry weight	28	1	100
Toasted Bran, Sainsbury	28	1	84
Toasted Crunchy Oats, Gateway	28	1	97
Toppas, Kellogg's	28	1	102
Weetabix, Weetabix	28	1	97
Weetaflake, Weetabix	28	1	99
Wheat Biscuits, Gateway	28	1	71
Wheat Flakes, Force	28	1	105
Wheatgerm, average	28	1	100
Wheat Honeys, Safeway	28	1	100
Wholewheat Bisks, Sainsbury	each		58
Wholewheat Flakes, Prewetts	28	1	92

		g	oz	Cal.

CONFECTIONERY
CHOCOLATE BARS

		g	oz	Cal.
Aero, Nestlé:				
milk	bar			252
mini		28	1	149
orange	bar			255
peppermint	bar			255
Animal Bar, Nestlé		28	1	150
Big Bar Bandit, McVitie's	each			215
Blue Riband, Nestlé	bar			116
Bounty, Mars, milk or plain	twin bar	57		276
Bournville Chocolate, Cadbury		28	1	142
Caramac, Nestlé, small	each			181
Chocolate Cream, Fry's	bar			210
Crunchie, Cadbury: treat size	bar			80
large	bar			195
Dairy Crunch Chocolate, Nestlé		32	1¼	162
Drifter, Nestlé	2 pieces			276
Galaxy Milk Chocolate, Mars, small		47		250

		g	oz	Cal.
Ginger Fudge, Carob coated snack, Kalibu	each			145
Golden Cup, Nestlé	small bar			102
Kit Kat, Nestlé	2-finger bar			109
	4-finger bar			245
Lion Bar, Nestlé	each			258
Mars Bar	bar	65		294
	Fun size bar	19		85
Milk Chocolate, Nestlé		28	1	150
Milk Chocolate Buttons, Boots		28	1	136
Milk Chocolate Waifa, Terry's	each			191
Milky Bar, Nestlé		28	1	153
Milky Way, Mars	each	26		117
	Fun size bar	17		74
Orange Cream, Cadbury	bar			210
Ovaltine Milk Chocolate, Wander	bar			255
Peppermint Cream, Fry's	small bar			208
Strollers, Cadbury, small	bar			105
Taxi, McVitie's	each			77
Toffee Crisp, Nestlé	each			243

	g	oz	Cal.
Topic, Mars	bar		239
Turkish Delight, Fry's	small bar		187
Twix, Mars	twin bar		272
Whole Nut Chocolate, Cadbury	bar		255
Yorkie, Nestlé:			
almond	each		325
milk	each		343
raisin & biscuit	each		284

CHOCOLATES

	g	oz	Cal.
After Eights, Nestlé	each		35
Chocolate Coated Peanuts, Tesco	28	1	151
Chocolate Whirls, Cadbury	each		130
Creme Eggs, Cadbury	each		175
Filled chocolates, average	28	1	130
Hazel Whirls, Cadbury	28	1	148
Maltesers, Mars	small bag	37 1½	183
Matchmakers, Nestlé	28	1	133

	g	oz	Cal.
Milk Chocolate Buttons, Sainsbury	28	1	136
Milk Chocolate Orange Segments, Terry's	whole		962
Milk Chocolate Toffee Roll, Callard & Bowser	each		38
Milk Tray Assortment, Cadbury	28	1	130
Mini Egg, Cadbury	bag		500
Minstrels, Mars	bag	42	1½	206
Mint Crisps, Elizabeth Shaw	each		30
Mint Leaves, Cadbury	28	1	126
Neapolitans, Terry's	195	7	1034
	each		30
Old Master Chocolate Liqueurs, Tobler Suchard	box 85	3	360
Orange Chocolate Eclairs, Callard & Bowser	each		32
Orange Crisps, Elizabeth Shaw	each		30
Plain Chocolate Orange, Terry's	whole		914
Praline Eclairs, Fry's	28	1	133
Quality Street, Nestlé	28	1	126

		g	oz	Cal.
Revels, Mars	small bag	35		173
Rolo, Nestlé	each			24
	pack			264
Roses Chocolate Assortment, Cadbury		28	1	134
Walnut Whip, Nestlé	each			169

HEALTH BARS

		g	oz	Cal.
Alpen Natural Crunch, Weetabix	each			115
Apple & Bran Health, Honeyrose	each			60
Apple & Date Dessert, Prewetts		28	1	72
Apple, Fruit & Nut, Shepherd Boy	each			150
Apple & Date Health Food, Granose	each			85
Banana Fruit, Prewetts		28	1	70
Banana Fruit & Nut Bar, Shepherd Boy	bar			150
Bran & Oat Crunch, Boots		28	1	85

		g	oz	Cal.
Carob Coated Country, Allinson	bar			151
Carob Coated Sesame, Allinson	bar			105
Carob Fruit, Granose	bar			144
Crunch, Carob Crunch, Kalibu	each			375
Crunchy Muesli & Raisin, Bisks	each			40
Crunchy Slice, Holly Mills	bar			187
Date & Fig Dessert, Prewetts	bar			142
Date & Muesli Bar, Boots	bar			155
Fruit, Kalibu		35	1¼	105
Fruit & Bran, Prewetts	bar			125
Fruit, Bran & Honey Crunch Bar, Sainsbury	each			140
Fruit & Nut, Honeyrose	each			100
Fruit & Nut Dessert, Prewetts	bar			130
Fruit & Nut Slice:				
Holly Mills	each			175
Sunpure	each			175
Ginger & Pear, Chocolate Coated, Boots	bar			150
Hazel Carob, Kalibu		42	1½	215

CONFECTIONERY

		g	oz	Cal.
Krunch, Carob Bar, Kalibu		75	2½	375
Mint Carob, Kalibu		28	1	106
	each			313
Nut Muesli, Carob coated, Kalibu	each	35	1¼	140
Oat, Apple & Almond:				
Holly Mills	bar			175
Sunpure	bar			175
Oat, Apple & Raisin:				
Holly Mills	bar			165
Sunpure	bar			165
Old Fashioned Honey & Muesli, Hornton's		50	2	110
Orange Carob, Kalibu	bar			313
Plain Carob, Kalibu	each			313
Roast Peanut, Holly Mills	each			155
Sesame Crunch: Allinson	each			115
Planters	each	40	1½	215
Sunflower Fruit & Nut, Shepherd Boy	each			190

		g	oz	Cal.

SWEETS, FUDGE AND GUMS

		g	oz	Cal.
Acid drops	each			20
Barley sugar, average		28	1	100
Boiled sweets, average		28	1	93
Butterscotch: average		28	1	115
Safeway	each			290
Butter Toffee Bon-bons, Fry's		28	1	108
Candy floss, average	stick			60
Cola Bottles, Trebor Bassett	each			10
Cough sweet, average: boiled	each			10
pastille	each			5
Curly Wurly, Cadbury	each			130
Dairy Fudge, Sharps	each			40
Dentyne Chewing Gum, all flavours	piece			5
Dessert Nougat, Callard & Bowser	each			62
Devon Toffee, Sainsbury		28	1	125
Dolly Mixtures: Bassett's		28	1	106
Sainsbury		113	4	412
St Michael		28	1	100

	g	oz	Cal.
Double Devon Toffee, St Michael	28	1	125
Doublemint Chewing Gum, Wrigley's each stick			10
Extra Strong Mint, Sharps each			10
Fox's Glacier Fruits, Nestlé each			20
Fox's Glacier Mints, Nestlé each			20
Fruit gum, average	28	1	50
Fruit pastilles, Nestlé carton			371
Fudge, average	28	1	110
Glitter Fruits, boiled, Trebor Bassett each			20
Golden Toffee, Nestlé	28	1	127
Hacks, all flavours, Fryers	28	1	100
Halva	28	1	125
Honey & Lemon, boiled sweets, Trebor each			20
Hubba Bubba, Wrigley's gum piece			15
Jelly Babies, Bassett's	28	1	92
Jellytots, Nestlé packet			153

		g	oz	Cal.
Jels, Green's	packet			135
Juicy Jellies, Callard & Bowser	each			30
Lemon Bon Bon, Sharps toffee	each			25
Lico-Jet, liquorice, Bassett's		28	1	81
Liquorice allsorts, average		28	1	105
Liquorice Comfits, Bassett's		28	1	101
Liquorice Novelties, Bassett's		28	1	82
Liquorice Toffee, Callard & Bowser	each			39
Little Big Feet, Trebor jellies	each			16
Lockets, Mars	small packet	43		165
Lollyade, Trebor Bassett	each			108
Marshmallows: average		28	1	90
Sainsbury		28	1	88
Menthol Stick Pack, Trebor Bassett	packet			125
Mini Allsorts, Sainsbury		28	1	94
Mint Lumps, Sainsbury		28	1	109
Mint Imperials, Maynards	bag			400
Mint Imperials, Sainsbury		28	1	104

		g	oz	Cal.
Mintoes, Callard & Bowser, loose	each			30
Mintola, Nestlé	pack			270
Mint Toffee, Callard & Bowser, loose	each			38
Mint Toffo, Nestlé	pack			202
Murray Mints, Pascall	each			25
Nougat: average		28	1	122
Terry's plain	each			45
Opal Fruits, Mars	bag	45.5		187
Pastilles, Callard & Bowser	each			9
Peanut Brittle, Trebor Bassett	each			42
Pear Drop, Trebor Bassett	each			16
Peppermints, average		28	1	110
Pink & White Marshmallows, Barker & Dobson		28	1	110
Polo Fruits, Nestlé	tube			109
Polo Mints, Nestlé	tube			102
Pontefract Cake, Bassett's		28	1	81
Popcorn, St Michael		28	1	119

FOOD

	g	oz	Cal.
Refresher, Trebor Bassett	tube			100
Rock: Edinburgh	stick			101
seaside	stick			90
Rolling Pin, Barratt	28	1	85
Rum & Raisin Fudge, Callard & Bowser	each			205
Sherbert Bon-bons, Barker & Dobson	28	1	100
Sherbert Dib Dabs, Barratt	28	1	99
Skittles, Mars	Fun size			91
Smarties, Nestlé	fun pack			67
	tube			173
Smith Kendon Travel Sweets, Callard & Bowser	each			20
Soft Crumbly Mints, St Michael	28	1	107
Spearmint Chewing Gum, Wrigley's	stick			10
Sugared Almonds, Terry's	each			19
Toasted Coconut Marshmallows, Barker & Dobson	28	1	108
Toffee Bon Bons, Sharps	each			30

		g	oz	Cal.
Toffees, average		28	1	122
Toffo, Nestlé	pack			211
Toffs, Callard & Bowser	each			49
Tunes, Mars, cherry or honey	packet			135
Turkish Delight, Terry's	each			41
Victory V Gums, Fryers		28	1	86
Victory V Lozenges, Fryers		28	1	95
Wine Gums: Bassett's		28	1	98
Fry's		28	1	97

DAIRY PRODUCTS

CHEESE AND CHEESE PRODUCTS

		g	oz	Cal.
Blue Brie		28	1	124
Boursin		28	1	115
Brie		28	1	85
Buxton Blue, Dairy Crest		28	1	118
Caerphilly		28	1	105

	g	oz	Cal.
Camembert	28	1	75
Cheddar	28	1	110
Cheddar, Mature, Cracker Barrel	28	1	115
Cheddar Slice, Kraft, processed	28	1	91
Cheddar with Walnut, Asda	28	1	115
Cheesies, Birds Eye	each		60
Cheshire	28	1	110
Cheviot	28	1	119
Cotswold	28	1	105
Cottage, Safeway	carton	340	354
Cream, Sainsbury	28	1	122
Curd	28	1	35
Danish Blue	28	1	100
Derby	28	1	113
Double Gloucester: with chives & onion, St Ivel	28	1	110
with pickled onion, beer & parsley, St Ivel	28	1	100
Dutch Gouda, Safeway	28	1	98
Edam	28	1	90

	g	oz	Cal.
Gorgonzola	28	1	112
Herb Roule, Safeway	28	1	100
Lancashire	28	1	101
Leicester, red	28	1	111
Lymeswold Cottage Cheese, Tesco	28	1	111
Mozzarella, grated, Sainsbury	28	1	70
Parmesan: average	28	1	120
Buitoni	28	1	142
Philadelphia Full Fat Soft, Kraft	28	1	88
Primula Cheese Spread, plain, Primula	28	1	71
Pont l'Évêque, St Michael	28	1	80
Port Salut	28	1	90
Processed Cheese Slices, Cheddar or Cheshire, Kraft	28	1	91
Quark	28	1	25
Roquefort	28	1	87
Somerset Goat's, Sainsbury	28	1	88
Stilton: average	28	1	115
white, Waitrose	28	1	98

	g	oz	Cal.
Swiss Knight Processed Gruyère	28	1	90
Tendale, Dairy Crest	28	1	72
Vignotte, Waitrose	28	1	134
Wensleydale	28	1	110
Yarg	28	1	108

EGGS

		g	oz	Cal.
Egg, average	size 1			95
	size 2			90
	size 3			85
	size 4			75
	size 5			70
	size 6			65
Duck egg, average	each	99	3½	170
Quail egg	each			15
Omelette, 3-egg with ham, average	each			250

	g	oz	Cal.

MILK AND MILK PRODUCTS

		g	oz	Cal.
Butter, average		28	I	220
	I tablespoon			105
Buttermilk	550ml/I pint			220
Aerosol Cream, Anchor	I tablespoon			5
Cream, average: clotted		28	I	165
Cornish		28	I	153
double		28	I	128
single, UHT		28	I	55
soured		28	I	54
tinned		28	I	70
whipped & compressed		28	I	105
whipping		28	I	105
Milk: semi-skimmed		600 ml	I pt	270
skimmed		600 ml	I pt	195
whole		600 ml	I pt	380
Quark		28	I	25

YOGHURT

		g	oz	Cal.
Apricot & Guava, St Michael	carton	100	3½	100
Apricot & Mango, Sainsbury	carton	150	5¼	176

		g	oz	Cal.
Apricot Mango Tropical, Eden Vale	carton	150	5¼	126
Black Cherry, St Michael		28	1	32
Bonjour, Chambourcy, all fruit flavours	carton	100	3½	85
Dennis the Menace, Dairy Crest, all flavours		125	4½	120
Diet, Very Low Fat, Yoplait	carton	125	4½	60
Drinking, fresh, Danish Quality Foods, Butterdane		500	17	350
French Recipe, Sainsbury		125	4½	100
Fruit, average		28	1	30
Fruit Corner, Müller		175	6	185
Frousse Raspberry & Cream, Ski	carton	150	5¼	152
Greek, Total, strained cow's milk	carton	450	14	608
Greek, Total, sheep's milk with cream	carton	450	14	470
Hazelnut: Co-op	carton	142	5	138
Loseley	carton	140	5	140
Ski	carton	150	5¼	149
Hazelnut, Sainsbury Low Fat	carton	150	5¼	150

		g	oz	Cal.
Jaffa, Mr Men, Raines	carton	125	4	125
Lebnie, Loseley	carton	145	5	170
Lemon Cheesecake, Safeway Low Fat	carton	125	4	63
Lunchbox, Anchor, all flavours	carton	100	3½	111
Mandarin Mousse, Co-op	carton	142	5	141
Melon & Ginger, Eden Vale	carton	125	4½	157
Mr Men, Sainsbury, average	carton	125	4½	110
Muesli, Loseley	carton	125	4½	150
Munch Bunch, strawberry, Eden Vale	carton	125	4½	106
Natural: Cool Country	carton	142	5	110
Eden Vale	carton	150	5¼	107
St Ivel	carton	125	4½	75
St Michael	carton	150	5¼	90
Natural Low Fat: Sainsbury	carton	450	14	270
Waitrose	carton	150	5¼	99
Passion Fruit & Melon, Eden Vale	carton	150	5¼	150
Pasteurised Fruit, Dairytime	carton	150	5¼	75
Pasteurised Natural, Dairytime	carton	150	5¼	145
Peach & Apricot, Sainsbury	carton	175	5¼	175

		g	oz	Cal.
Peach Melba: Dairytime	carton	120	4½	105
Mr Men	carton	150	5¼	140
St Ivel		28	1	12
Peach & Praline, Chambourcy	carton	142	5	95
Peach & Papaya, Co-op	carton	142	5	164
Pear & Banana, Dessert Farm	carton	142	5	87
Pear Melba, Ski	carton	150	5¼	108
Pineapple & Coconut, Eden Vale	carton	150	5¼	150
Plum, Boots, Custard Style	carton	175	6	209
Prize Black Cherry Fruit, St Ivel	carton	142	5	90
Rhubarb, Sainsbury, Low Fat	carton	150	5¼	140
Strawberry, Mr Men, Raines	carton	125	4	115
Tropical Fruit, Safeway	carton	150	5¼	150
Vanilla, Eden Vale	carton	150	5¼	138
Whole Milk Black Cherry, St Michael	carton	150	5¼	163
Wholemilk Natural Set, Safeway		28	1	25

	g	oz	Cal.

DIABETIC

	g	oz	Cal.
Apricot Jam, Country Preserves	28	1	35
Hazelnut Milk Chocolate, Boots	28	1	138
Jelly, Boots	tablet		240
Lemon Curd, Ratcliffe	28	1	95
Milk Chocolate, Boots	28	1	128
Orange Flavour Milk Chocolate, Boots	28	1	128
Pastilles, all flavours, Boots	28	1	66
Plain Chocolate, Boots	28	1	129
Raspberry Jam:			
Country Preserves	28	1	35
Whole Earth	28	1	35
Strawberry Jam, Country Preserves	28	1	35
Threeberry Jam, Country Preserves	28	1	41

		g	oz	Cal.

DRIED AND GLACÉ FRUIT AND NUTS

		g	oz	Cal.
Almonds: flaked	1 tablespoon			40
whole, Princess, Barker & Dobson		28	1	127
Apricots: average		28	1	52
Beddingtons Fruit Company	packet	142	4	195
Banana Chips, Tesco		28	1	145
Barcelona nuts, shelled, average		28	1	183
Beechnuts, shelled, average		28	1	160
Big D Tropical Fruit & Nuts, Smiths	packet	50	1¾	175
Brazil nuts, average:				
chocolate coated	each			55
shelled		28	1	75
Brazil Kernels, Sainsbury		28	1	175
Cashew nuts: dry roasted		28	1	129
shelled, plain		28	1	178
Cashew nuts, salted, Tesco		28	1	165
Cherry, glacé		28	1	60

		g	oz	Cal.
Chestnuts: purée, average	tinned	28	1	65
shelled		28	1	48
Chopped Mixed Fruit, Whitworth's		28	1	160
Cob nuts: shelled		28	1	28
weighed with shells		28	1	39
Coconut: creamed		28	1	218
desiccated, average		28	1	171
fresh		28	1	102
Currants, average, dried		28	1	69
Date & Cashew Muesli Tub, Jordans	each			26
Dates: chopped & sugar rolled, average		28	1	77
chopped & sugar rolled, Whitworth's		28	1	73
dried, without stone, average		28	1	70
dried with stone, average		28	1	60
stoned, Whitworth's		28	1	30
Doublenut Mix: Granny Smith	packet			820
Lyons Tetley	packet			880
Dry Roasted Peanuts:				
KP	packet	50	2	295
Planters	packet	50	2	285

FOOD

		g	oz	Cal.
Sainsbury	packet	100	3½	590
Walker's	packet	50	2	265
Figs, average		28	1	60
Ginger stem in syrup, average		28	1	60
Hazelnuts, shelled, average		28	1	108
Macedonia nuts, shelled, average		28	1	187
Marrons glacés		28	1	75
Mixed nuts & raisins: average		28	1	151
Smiths		50	2	185
Mixed peel, candied		28	1	78
Nutmeg				0
Nuts & Raisins, Golden Wonder		28	1	150
Pancho Peanuts, Trebor Bassett	each			5
Pancho Raisins, Trebor Bassett	each			5
Peach: average		28	1	61
stewed without sugar		28	1	20
Peanuts, average:				
dry roasted		28	1	171
roasted & salted		28	1	162
Peanuts & Raisins, KP		100		443
Pear, average		28	1	45
Pecan nuts, average		28	1	150

	g	oz	Cal.
Pine kernels	28	1	180
Pistachio nuts: weighed with shells, average	28	1	168
St Michael	28	1	177
Prunes: No-need-to-soak, Whitworth's	28	1	30
uncooked, weighed whole	28	1	38
Pumpkin seeds	28	1	180
Raisins, average	28	1	70
Roast Salted Peanuts, KP	25	¾	150
Salted Cashew Nuts, Sainsbury	50	2	320
Salted Peanuts, Golden Wonder packet			50
Sesame seeds	28	1	168
Sultanas, dried, average	28	1	71
Sunflower seed, skinned	28	1	170
Sweet Almonds, Whitworth's	28	1	160
Sweet Peanuts, Trebor Bassett each			25
Walnuts: pickled, Epicure	28	1	20
shelled, Sun-Pat	28	1	147
with shells	28	1	100
Water Chestnuts, Amoy tinned	283	10	104

	g	oz	Cal.

FATS AND OILS

		g	oz	Cal.
Butter, average		28	1	205
Cod liver oil	1 teaspoon			40
Dripping		28	1	250
	per tablespoon/15ml			125
Flora		28	1	210
Ghee		28	1	235
Gold, Standard or Unsalted, St Ivel		28	1	111
Golden Churn Spread, Kraft		28	1	182
Kerrygold Lite Spread, Kerrygold		28	1	110
Krona Spreadable		28	1	59
Lard		28	1	250
Low Fat Spread, Safeway		28	1	101
Margarine, average		28	1	226
Oil:	per tablespoon/15ml			125
corn		28	1	255
ground nut		28	1	255
olive		28	1	255
soya bean		28	1	255

	g	oz	Cal.
sunflower	28	1	255
vegetable	28	1	255
Outline Very Low Fat Spread, van der Burgh	28	1	73
Slimmers' Spread, Co-op	28	1	105
Stork Light Blend	28	1	153
Suet: block	28	1	255
shredded	28	1	235
dumpling mix, Granny Smith	packet		1130
pudding mix, Lyons Tetley	packet		1120
Sunflower Low Fat Spread	28	1	110

FISH

	g	oz	Cal.
Bass, average steamed fillet	28	1	35
Bloater, average, grilled, weighed with skin & bones	28	1	53
Catfish, steamed with bones	28	1	28
Caviar, average	28	1	75
Clam, raw without shell	28	1	25
Cockle, boiled without shell	28	1	15

FOOD

	g	oz	Cal.
Cod: baked or steamed	28	1	23
fried in batter	28	1	57
Cod's roe	28	1	32
Coley, fillet, steamed	28	1	28
Crab: meat only, boiled	28	1	37
weighed with shell	28	1	7
Prince's	28	1	25
Eel: jellied	28	1	60
raw, flesh only	28	1	50
smoked	28	1	56
Flounder, steamed with bones	28	1	15
Haddock: fried with skin & bones	28	1	21
smoked, steamed with skin & bones	28	1	28
Hake: fried, weighed with skin & bones	28	1	55
steamed, weighed with skin & bones	28	1	24
Halibut, steamed with skin & bones	28	1	28
Herring: baked in vinegar, weighed with skin & bones	28	1	50

	g	oz	Cal.
fried, weighed with skin & bones	28	1	59
roe, raw	28	1	23
John Dory, steamed, weighed with skin & bones	28	1	17
Kipper: grilled or baked	28	1	31
raw	28	1	45
Ling, fried, weighed with skin & bones	28	1	52
Lobster:			
weighed, meat only, cooked	28	1	34
weighed with shell, cooked	28	1	12
Mackerel:			
fried, weighed with skin & bones	28	1	39
kippered, weighed with skin & bones	28	1	70
raw, weighed with skin & bones	28	1	40
smoked, weighed with skin & bones	28	1	68
Monkfish:			
fried, weighed with skin & bones	28	1	41
steamed, weighed with skin & bones	28	1	23

FOOD

	g	oz	Cal.
Mullet, red or grey, steamed, weighed with skin & bones	28	1	23
Mussels:			
boiled	28	1	25
boiled, weighed with shells	28	1	7
Octopus, raw	28	1	20
Oysters, raw: without shells	28	1	15
with shells	28	1	2
Perch, raw, weighed whole	28	1	35
Pike, raw, weighed whole	28	1	25
Plaice: raw	28	1	26
steamed, weighed with skin & bones	28	1	14
Pollan: fried in oatmeal	28	1	40
steamed, weighed with skin & bones	28	1	16
Pollock, raw, weighed with skin & bones	28	1	25
Prawns: shelled	28	1	30
with shells	28	1	12
Saithe: steamed	28	1	28
steamed & weighed whole	28	1	24

		g	oz	Cal.
Salmon:				
boiled or steamed		28	1	56
boiled or steamed, weighed				
with skin & bones		28	1	45
raw		28	1	52
smoked		28	1	40
Salmon trout: raw, flesh only		28	1	50
boiled or				
steamed		28	1	54
Sardines, raw		28	1	55
Scallops: raw		28	1	20
steamed without shells		28	1	30
Scampi, raw, peeled		28	1	30
Shark, raw, flesh only		28	1	50
Shrimps: fresh, peeled		28	1	33
fresh with shells		28	1	11
drained, average	tinned	28	1	27
John West	tinned	100	3½	90
Skate, fillet, fried in batter		28	1	57
Smelt, boneless, fried		28	1	115
Sole, Dover fillet:				
fried		28	1	61
raw		28	1	23
steamed or poached,				
weighed whole		28	1	18

	g	oz	Cal.
Sole, lemon, whole, poached	28	1	18
Sprats, fried	28	1	110
Squid, raw	28	1	25
Sturgeon, raw, weighed with bones	28	1	25
Trout, weighed whole:			
poached or grilled	28	1	20
smoked	28	1	21
Turbot, fillet, poached	28	1	28
Whelks, weighed with shells	28	1	4
Whitebait, fried	28	1	152
Whiting:			
fried, weighed whole	28	1	49
steamed, weighed whole	28	1	17
Winkles, steamed or boiled, weighed with shells	28	1	4
Witch:			
fried, weighed whole	28	1	56
steamed, weighed whole	28	1	15

	g	oz	Cal.

FISH DISHES

	g	oz	Cal.
Baked Herrings, Waitrose	28	1	54
Battercrisp Jumbo Cod Chunks, Ross	28	1	50
Battered Crisp Cod Portions, Birds Eye	28	1	55
Battered Crispy Cod, Ross	28	1	57
Battered Cod Steak, Birds Eye	each		230
Buttered Kipper Fillet, Young's	28	1	54
Buttered Smoked Haddock, Young's	100	3½	82
Captain's Pie, Birds Eye	pack		315
Cod Crumble, Ross	28	1	50
Cod in Breadcrumbs, Safeway	28	1	62
Cod in Butter Sauce, Birds Eye	packet		160
Cod in Cheese Sauce, Birds Eye	packet		170
Cod with Parsley Sauce, Tesco	28	1	23
Cod Fish Finger, Birds Eye	each		50
Cod & Prawn Pie, St Michael	28	1	47

		g	oz	Cal.
Cod Steak in Crisp Crunch Crumbs, Birds Eye	each			220
Cod's roe, average, fried in egg & breadcrumbs		28	1	55
Cod Steak in Parsley Sauce, Birds Eye	packet			155
Coley Fillet, Co-op		28	1	22
Cordon Bleu Fish, Iceland	portion			300
Crispy Plaice Fillet, Birds Eye		28	1	60
Cumberland Fish Pie, St Michael		28	1	35
Dressed Crab, John West	tinned	45	1½	60
Economy Cod Fish Fingers, Findus, grilled	each			63
Fishburger, Birds Eye, baked (Captain's Quarter Pounder)	each			245
Fish Cake:				
average, fried		28	1	53
average, grilled	each			65
Co-op, grilled	each			157
Fish Finger:				
average, fried		28	1	65
average grilled	each			50

	g	oz	Cal.
Ross, grilled	28	1	51
St Michael	454	16	615
Fish pie, average	28	1	36
Fish Steak in Butter Sauce, Ross	28	1	26
Fish Stick, Ocean Pearl	each		15
Fish & Chips, Wimpy	portion		465
Haddock:			
in batter, Safeway	28	1	63
in Crisp Crunch Crumbs, Birds Eye	each		220
fillets, breaded and frozen, Waitrose	28	1	54
smoked with butter, Birds Eye	28	1	26
smoked fillet with butter, Iceland	28	1	27
steaks in butter sauce, Ross	28	1	26
Haddock Fish Finger, Findus, grilled	each		63
Haddock Mornay, St Michael	400	14	440
Haddock Steak in Light Crispy Crumb, Findus	packet		250

		g	oz	Cal.
Haddock Steaklet in Crunchy Crumb, Findus		28	1	60
Herring:				
fillets in savoury sauce, John West	tinned	200	7	265
fillets in tomato sauce, John West	tinned	200	7	410
roe, fried		28	1	70
Jumbo Cod Fingers, Ross		28	1	69
Kedgeree, average		28	1	43
Kipper:				
fillets in oil, Prince's	tinned	190	7	565
fillets, John West	tinned	200	7½	452
Kippered Mackerel Fillets, Macrae	tinned	28	1	55
Mackerel in Brine, Sainsbury	tinned	125	4	238
Mackerel Fillets in Oil, Prince's	tinned	125	4	272
Mackerel in Tomato Sauce, Prince's	tinned	125	4	276
Mariners Bake, St Michael		28	1	30
North Atlantic Prawns, Safeway, frozen		100	3½	107

		g	oz	Cal.
Ocean Pie: Ross		28	1	33
St Michael	packet	227	8	240
Oven Crispy Cod Steak:				
Birds Eye, as sold	each			230
baked or grilled	each			215
Oven Crispy Fish Finger, Birds Eye	each			80
Oven Crispy Haddock Steak:				
Birds Eye, as sold	each			230
baked or grilled	each			215
Paella, Vesta, serves 2	packet			640
Pilchards:				
tinned & drained of oil, average		28	1	54
tinned in tomato sauce, average		28	1	36
tinned in tomato sauce, John West		425	15	550
tinned in tomato sauce, Prince's		227	8	345
Pink Salmon, John West	tinned	105	3½	163
Plaice:				
fillets, breaded, St Michael	packet	454	1 lb	415
fillets, frozen, Waitrose		28	1	25
Florentine, St Michael		28	1	38
fried in batter, average		28	1	40

		g	oz	Cal.
steaks in Crispy Crunch Crumb, Birds Eye	each			200
whole, battered, grilled, Findus		28	1	34
Prawn Cocktail Goblet, Mattessons		100	3½	197
Prawn Curry: Chic-o-Roll	packet	170	6	104
Vesta, serves 2	packet			730
Prawn Curry with Rice, Findus	per serving	300		276
Prawns, peeled, Armour	tinned	200	7	192
Pressed Cod's Roe, John West	tinned	200	7	210
Red Salmon, John West, drained	tinned	105	3½	165
Salmon: average	tinned	28	1	44
red, Sainsbury	tinned	212	7½	350
Salmon Fish Cake:				
fried, average	each			160
grilled without fat, Birds Eye	each			90
Salmon pâté, average		28	1	60
Sardine:				
in brine, John West	tinned	120	4½	215
in oil drained, average	tinned	28	1	62
in oil, John West	tinned	120	4½	255

		g	oz	Cal.
in oil, Prince's	tinned	120	4½	415
in tomato sauce, John West	tinned	120	4½	280
Savoury Fish Cake, Birds Eye:				
fried	each			150
grilled without fat	each			65
Scampi:				
breaded, as sold, Presto		28	– 1	40
Thermidor with Rice,				
Baxters	tinned	312	11	360
Sild in Oil, Gateway	tinned	100	3½	380
Smoked Haddock with butter,				
Findus	packet	170	6	170
Smoked Mackerel fillets in oil,				
drained, John West	tinned	110	4 –	340
Smoked Trout Pâté, Tesco		28	1	72
Taramasalata, average		28	1	130
Tuna:				
in brine & drained, average	tinned	28	1	31
in brine, John West	tinned	100	3½	110
in brine, Sainsbury	tinned	198	7	238
in oil & drained, average	tinned	28	1	62
in oil & drained, Prince's	tinned	100	3½	197
Tuna & Mushroom, Tiffany's				
'Upper Crust'	pack			1700

		g	oz	Cal.
Tuna in Curry Sauce,				
John West	tinned	185	6½	255
Value Cod Fish Finger, frozen,				
Gateway	each			52
Value Fish Finger, grilled,				
Birds Eye	each			45

FRUIT

		g	oz	Cal.
Apple: baked without sugar		28	1	11
cooking, raw		28	1	11
eating, skin & core		28	1	10
eating, whole, average		28	1	9
stewed with sugar		28	1	18
Apricot Halves in Fruit Juice,				
Sainsbury	tinned	411	14½	123
Apricot:				
raw, fresh, weighed with				
stones		28	1	7
	each			25
stewed without sugar				
or stones		28	1	35
stewed with sugar		28	1	19
Banana		28	1	23

		g	oz	Cal.
Blackberries:				
raw, fresh, frozen		28	1	8
stewed without sugar		28	1	7
Blackcurrants:				
Hartley's	tinned	284	10	102
raw, fresh, frozen, average		28	1	8
stewed without sugar		28	1	7
tinned in syrup		28	1	23
Boysenberry, Libby	tinned	28	1	19
Cherry, average:				
cocktail	each			10
fresh, weighed with stones		28	1	11
tinned		28	1	20
Cranberries, raw		28	1	4
Damson:				
fresh with stones		28	1	11
stewed with stones, no sugar		28	1	8
Date, fresh with stone	each	28	1	30
Fruit Cocktail:				
Armour	tinned	425	15	405
average	tinned	28	1	26
in apple juice, Koo	tinned	227	8	90
in apple juice, Libby's	tinned	411	14½	214
in apple juice, Waitrose	tinned	205	7	100

		g	oz	Cal.
Fruit Salad: Del Monte	tinned	227	8	152
John West	tinned	285	10	145
average	tinned	28	1	26
Armour		425	15	405
Ginger stem in syrup, average		28	1	60
Gooseberries:				
green, raw		28	1	5
stewed with sugar		28	1	14
Asda	tinned	283	10	80
Hartley's	tinned	283	10	175
Grapes: black, whole		28	1	14
white, whole		28	1	17
Grapefruit, whole fruit weighed		28	1	3
Grapefruit Segments:				
John West	tinned	285	10	80
Prince's	tinned	285	10	92
Tesco, in natural juices	tinned	220		81
Greengage:				
raw		28	1	13
stewed with sugar, weighed				
with stones		28	1	20
Guava: fresh		28	1	16
average	tinned	28	1	17
Kiwi fruit: fresh	each			30
Libby	tinned	28	1	19

	g	oz	Cal.
Lemon: juice			0
whole	28	1	4
Loganberries:			
fresh	28	1	5
in natural juice, John West tinned	285	10	105
in syrup, average	28	1	29
Lychee: fresh each			8
average tinned	28	1	19
in syrup, Safeway tinned	28	1	25
Mandarin:			
average tinned	28	1	18
fresh, weighed with skin			
& pips	28	1	7
in natural juices, John West tinned	28	1	13
Mandarin Oranges in syrup,			
John West tinned	298	10½	150
Mango: raw, flesh only	28	1	17
slices, Sainsbury	28	1	20
Medlar, weighed whole	28	1	10
Melon: canteloupe, whole	28	1	4
charentais, whole	28	1	3
honeydew, whole	28	1	4
Ogen, whole	28	1	5
yellow, whole	28	1	4
seeds	28	1	160
watermelon, whole	28	1	2

FOOD

		g	oz	Cal.
Mulberries, raw		28	1	10
Nectarine, weighed with stone		28	1	13
Olives:				
with stones in brine		28	1	23
without stones in brine		28	1	29
stuffed	each			5
Orange: flesh		28	1	10
skin, pips		28	1	7½
weighed with skin		28	1	7
whole fruit, small		140	5	35
Passion fruit, weighed whole		28	1	4
Paw-paw, fresh, flesh only		28	1	11
	tinned	28	1	19
Peach:				
fresh, weighed with stone		28	1	9
tinned, in natural juices, average		28	1	13
tinned, in syrup, average		28	1	25
Prince's, in juice	tinned	411	14½	205
Peach Halves or Slices in fruit juice, Del Monte	tinned	411	14½	197
Pear:				
in apple juice, Waitrose	tinned	205	7	72
in natural juice, average	tinned	28	1	11
raw, weighed whole		28	1	9

		g	oz	Cal.
in syrup, average		28	1	22
in syrup, Safeway	tinned	425	15	327
stewed, without sugar		28	1	8
Pear Halves:				
in apple juice, Koo	tinned	227	8	103
in fruit juice, Del Monte	tinned	227	8	114
Pear Quarters in Natural Juice, Sainsbury	tinned	285	10	100
Pineapple:				
fresh, weighed without skin		28	1	13
in natural juice, average	tinned	28	1	15
in syrup, average	tinned	28	1	22
Pineapple Slices:				
in syrup, Del Monte	tinned	234	8	183
in natural juice, Sainsbury	tinned	227	8	136
Pineapple Titbits, Libby's	tinned	411	14½	206
Plum:				
cooking, weighed with stones		28	1	7
Smedley's	tinned	540	19	430
Victoria, weighed with stones		28	1	10
Pomegranate: flesh only		28	1	20
juice		28	1	13
Prune:				
in light syrup, Hartley's	tinned	210	7½	233

		g	oz	Cal.
ready cooked, Whitworth's	dried	28	1	30
stewed without sugar, weighed whole		28	1	19
in natural juice, Safeway	tinned	220	7½	262
Pumpkin, raw, flesh only		28	1	4
Quinces		28	1	7
Raspberries:				
average		28	1	7
average	tinned	28	1	25
in juice, Co-op	tinned	220	7½	65
in syrup, Sainsbury		28	1	22
Redcurrants:				
raw		28	1	6
stewed without sugar		28	1	4
Rhubarb:				
Sainsbury	tinned	538	19	162
stewed without sugar		28	1	2
Satsuma, weighed whole	each	70	2½	20
Strawberries:				
fresh		28	1	7
Fruit Fruitfull, Beddington's	packet	142	5	180
Hartley's	tinned	284	10	207
in syrup, Safeway	tinned	312	11	255
in syrup, Sainsbury	tinned	370	13	240
drained, average	tinned	28	1	23

	g	oz	Cal.
Tangerine, weighed whole	28	1	9
Tropical Fruits, St Michael	28	1	15
White currants, stewed without sugar	28	1	6

HERBS, SPICES AND BASICS

	g	oz	Cal.
Arrowroot	28	1	100
Bovril Cubes	each		10
Brown Sugar Teamates, Patersons	each		60
Caper	28	1	5
Carob powder	28	1	50
Chilli: dried	28	1	85
fresh	28	1	6
Chive	28	1	10
Couscous, Waitrose	28	1	66
Curry paste, average	28	1	42
Curry powder, average	28	1	66
Gelatine	28	1	95
Ginger: ground	28	1	72
root, peeled	28	1	18

	g	oz	Cal.
Glucose, liquid, BP	28	1	90
Grenadine syrup	28	1	72
Gherkin	28	1	5
Horseradish:			
creamed, Gateway	28	1	47
hot, Burgess	28	1	58
raw	28	1	17
relish, Colman	28	1	28
Hot Chilli Sauce, Sharwood	28	1	34
Houmous: average	28	1	50
St Michael	227	8	626
Lentils: brown, boiled	28	1	32
brown, uncooked	28	1	104
red, boiled	28	1	28
red, uncooked	28	1	86
Malt extract, average	28	1	86
Marmite	28	1	2
Mild Curry Paste, Sharwood	28	1	100
Mint Jelly, Pearce Duff	28	1	74
Mustard Powder:			
average	28	1	132
Colmans made up	28	1	50
Natex Low Salt Savoury Spread, Modern Health Products	28	1	60
Nutmeg			0

		g	oz	Cal.
Olive: with stone in brine		28	1	23
without stone in brine		28	1	29
stuffed	each			5
stuffed, Crosse & Blackwell		28	1	15
Oxo Cube, average	each			16
Pepper, all kinds				0
Pumpkin seeds		28	1	180
Salt				0
Sesame seeds		28	1	168
Sugar: brown, caster, Demerara, granulated, icing & white		28	1	112
lump: large	each			20
small	each			10
Sunflower seeds, skinned		28	1	170
Tomato Purée: average		28	1	20
Sainsbury	jar	312	11	312
Vanilla essence		28	1	0
Vegetable Cube, Knorr Stock Cube		28	1	90
Vindaloo Curry Sauce, Sharwood's Goan	tinned	283	10	249

		g	oz	Cal.
Vinegar	1 tablespoon			½
Virol		28	1	99
Yeast Extract, Natex		28	1	70
Yeast: dried		28	1	48
fresh		28	1	15

JAMS, PRESERVES AND PICKLES

	g	oz	Cal.
Barbecue Relish, Co-op	28	1	26
Beetroot Pickle:			
Baxter's	28	1	10
Epicure, sweet, sliced	28	1	13
Beetroot & Redcurrant Relish, Baxter's	28	1	47
Branston Pickle, Crosse & Blackwell	28	1	42
Chutney:			
average, apple	28	1	57
average, tomato	28	1	43
average, mango	28	1	120
mango, Burgess	28	1	60

	g	oz	Cal.
mango & ginger, Green			
Label, Sharwood	28	1	61
peach, Sharwood	28	1	46
Extra Jams, all flavours, Chivers	28	1	71
Golden Syrup, average	1 tablespoon		60
Honey, average	28	1	90
Honeycomb	28	1	80
Jam, average:			
made with edible seeds	28	1	60
made with stone fruit	28	1	60
Lemon Cheese, Hartley's	28	1	85
Lemon Curd: average	28	1	80
Chivers	28	1	80
Gales	28	1	79
Malaysian Mild Curry Paste,			
Sharwood	28	1	65
Mango Chutney, Pan-Yan	28	1	77
Marmalade:			
average, home-made	28	1	74
Country Basket, no sugar	28	1	32
Frank Cooper Oxford			
Coarse Cut	28	1	74
Roses	28	1	75

	g	oz	Cal.
Mayonnaise: average	28	1	205
Burgess	28	1	172
Hellmann's	28	1	202
Mild Chilli Relish, Bicks	28	1	26
Mixed Pickles, Haywards	28	1	2
Mustard Piccalilli, Asda	28	1	13
Peach Chutney, Waitrose	28	1	52
Piccalilli:			
Hayward's	28	1	8
Heinz, Ploughmans	28	1	25
Pickled Jalapenos, Old El Paso	28	1	8
Pickled Silverskin Onions:			
average	each		5
Epicure	28	1	4
Sweet, Epicure	28	1	7
Pickled Gherkins, Epicure	28	1	5
Pickled Sliced Beetroot, Epicure	28	1	15
Pickled Walnuts, Epicure	28	1	22
Ploughmans Pickle, Heinz	28	1	33
Sweetcorn Relish, Presto	28	1	32

	g	oz	Cal.
Sweet Military Pickle, Hayward's	28	1	37
Sweet Pickle, Happy Farm	28	1	38
Sweet Pickled Onions, Co-op	28	1	45
Tomato & Chilli Relish, Sainsbury	28	1	45
Tomato Chutney, Baxter's	28	1	41
Tomato Pickle, Heinz	28	1	28
Tomato Relish: Burgess	28	1	31
Crosse & Blackwell	28	1	42
Wild Bramble Jelly, Baxter's	28	1	56

MEAT

		g	oz	Cal.
Bacon:				
collar joint, boiled, lean & fat		28	1	92
grilled well, average	rasher	30—35	1—1¼	80
streaky, grilled or fried	rasher	20	¾	50
Beef:				
brisket, boiled		28	1	90
fillet steak, grilled		175	6	250

	g	oz	Cal.
minced beef, raw	28	1	65
minced beef, fried in oil, drained of fat	28	1	80
rump steak: fried & trimmed	28	1	54
well grilled, raw weight	175	6	260
grilled rare, raw weight	175	6	310
silverside, boiled	28	1	69
sirloin, roasted	28	1	80
stewing steak: braised	28	1	65
raw	28	1	50
topside: raw	28	1	53
roasted	28	1	62
Brains: calf's, boiled	28	1	43
lamb's, boiled	28	1	36
Brawn	28	1	43
Gammon, boiled:			
lean & fat	28	1	91
lean only	28	1	54
Gammon rashers:			
fried: back, lean & fat	28	1	121
streaky, lean & fat	28	1	138
grilled: back, lean & fat	28	1	113
streaky, lean & fat	28	1	118
Hare: roast	28	1	55
stewed or baked	28	1	54

	g	oz	Cal.
Heart, sheep's	28	1	68
Kidney: ox, stewed	28	1	45
sheep, fried	28	1	33
Lamb:			
leg: lean & fat without bone	28	1	68
roast, lean & fat without bone	28	L	75
loin chop, grilled, average size			160
stewing, lean & fat without bone	28	1	72
Liver:			
calf's: fried	28	1	72
uncooked	28	1	43
chicken: fried	28	1	55
uncooked	28	1	38
lamb's: fried	28	1	66
raw	28	1	51
ox, stewed	28	1	55
pig's, raw	28	1	44
Oxtail:			
stewed & weighed with bones	28	1	25
stewed & weighed without bones	28	1	70
Ox tongue, boiled & pressed	28	1	35

FOOD

	g	oz	Cal.
Pork:			
chop, grilled, lean & fat, weighed whole	28	1	73
leg, roast, lean & fat	28	1	90
loin, roast, lean only	28	1	81
shoulder, St Michael chilled meats	28	1	36
Rabbit, stewed, weighed with bones	28	1	26
Silverside, Mattessons	28	1	50
Snails	28	1	25
Sweetbreads, lamb: fried	28	1	65
raw	28	1	37
Tripe, stewed	28	1	28
Veal: fillet, roast	28	1	65
escalope, fried	28	1	61
Venison, roast	28	1	56

MEAT DISHES

		g	oz	Cal.
Bacon Topper with Cheese, St Michael		28	1	82
Beef Chow Mein, Batchelor's Snack Pot	pack	230		145

		g	oz	Cal.
Beef Curry, Vesta, cooked	2-serving packet			958
Beef Curry with Rice, Birds Eye Menu Master	packet			395
Beef Grill Steak, Ross		28	1	88
Beef & Onion, Tesco		198	7	329
Beef Madras & Rice, Boots	pack			350
Beef Stew, Campbells	tinned	425	15	270
Beef Stew & Dumplings, Birds Eye Menu Master	packet			350
Boeuf Bourguignon, Baxters	tinned	440	15½	431
Braised Steak in Rich Gravy, St Michael		28	1	24
Breaded Chicken Kiev, Ross		28	1	67
Chicken Breast with Yoghurt & Mint, St Michael		28	1	44
Chicken Madras, Shippams		28	1	24
Chilli Con Carne, St Michael		28	1	32
Corned Beef Hash: Tiffany	tin			185
Sharwoods	each			168
Cottage pie, average		28	1	89
Dinner Balls, Granose	tinned	100	3½	145

	g	oz	Cal.
Doner kebab, average	each			550
Faggots:			
average	28	1	75
Brains, in rich sauce	28	1	40
Faggots with onions in rich sauce, Ross	100	3½	160
Gammon-Style Turkey Steak, grilled, Matthew's	28	1	52
Gravy with Sliced Beef, Ross	100	3½	61
Hash Browns, frozen, Ross	28	1	23
Haggis, cooked, average	28	1	88
Hot Dogs, Wall's, tinned	each		60
Hot Dogs, mini, Tesco	tinned	28	1	60
International Grill, Wimpy	portion			730
Irish Stew: Newforge	tinned	400	14	255
Tyne Brand	tinned	392	14	320
Kashmir Beef Curry, Knorr	100		83
Lamb Casserole, St Michael	100	3½	110
Lamb Dalesteak, grilled, Dalepak	each	85	3	200
Liver with Onion & Gravy, Birds Eye Menu Master Meal	pack			150

		g	oz	Cal.
London Grill, Crosse & Blackwell Ready Meal		283	10	359
Meatballs:				
Danepak, fresh	each			32
in gravy, Campbells		410	14½	332
in tomato sauce, Campbells		410	14½	357
Mexican Style Chilli Beef Roll, Plumrose		28	1	54
Mince, Baxters, Scotch		432	15½	415
Mince Bolognese, Tyne Brand	tinned	412	14½	490
Minced Beef & Onion in gravy, Co-op	tinned	425	15	690
St Michael	tinned	28	1	47
Minced Beef & Vegetable Bake, Safeway, frozen	each	100	3½	106
Norfolk Burger, Bernard Matthews		28	1	59
Pork & Beef Sausage, Cotswold Style	each			120
Pork Dalesteak, Dalepak, well grilled	each			180
Pork Roll with Egg, Tesco		28	1	76
Roast Beef in Gravy, Findus		100	3½	84

		g	oz	Cal.
Roast Turkey in Gravy, Birds Eye, frozen	pack			220
Rogan Josh: Chic-o-Roll	packet	170	6	150
Homepride	tinned			380
Sausage:				
beef: chipolata, well grilled	each			50
large, well grilled	each			120
skinless, well grilled	each			65
Waitrose		28	1	72
pork: boiling ring		28	1	110
chipolata, well grilled	each			65
large, well grilled	each			125
skinless, well grilled	each			95
Wall's, Best English	each	28	1	93
pork & beef: chipolata, well grilled	each			60
large, well grilled	each			125
turkey & pork: Matthew's, grilled	each			160
Sausage meat, uncooked		28	1	80
Savoury Pudding, Granose	tinned	454	16	940
Savoury Soufflé, Daloon	pack			610
Shepherd's pie		100	3½	250
Spare Ribs in Barbecue Sauce:				
Chic-o-Roll		227	8	410
Mr Chang	packet	227	8	420

		g	oz	Cal.
Stewed Steak, Prince's	tinned	28	1	31
Stewpot, Ross, Beef & Kidney	each			495
Sweet & Sour Chicken with Rice, Birds Eye	packet			385
Sweet & Sour Pork with Vegetables, Uncle Wong's		283	10	440
Toad-in-the-hole, average		225	8	500
Wimpy Grill, Wimpy	each			218

MICROWAVE DISHES

		g	oz	Cal.
Beef Bolognese, Crosse & Blackwell		28	1	90
Beef Bourguignon, Ross Micro-Cook		28	1	25
Beef Casserole, Batchelor's Microchef	pack			240
Broad Beans, Froqual, Microwave		28	1	14
Cantonese Sweet & Sour Pork, Sharwood		28	1	46
Chop Suey, Uncle Ben Sauce		28	1	19

	g	oz	Cal.
Coffee Gâteau, Green's Microwave Magic	28	1	85
Creamy Herb Fish, Colman Cuisine	28	1	115
Gammon Hawaii, Crosse & Blackwell	28	1	100
Hamburger in a Bun, Iceland	each		350
Ham & Mushroom Tagliatelle, Batchelor's	each		310
Indian Beef Curry, Wilson	28	1	57
Indian Chicken Korma, Campbells	28	1	46
Lamb Hotpot, Boots	each		141
Lasagne, Safeway	28	1	45
Malaysian Chicken Satay, Sharwood	28	1	40
Microwave Crumble, Homepride	28	1	133
Peking Barbecue Spare Ribs, Knorr	28	1	25
Rogan Josh, Co-op	28	1	35
Seafood Tagliatelle, John West	28	1	30

	g	oz	Cal.
Sweet & Sour Pork, Crosse & Blackwell	28	1	100
Syrup Pudding, Homepride Microbake	28	1	92
Tomato & Cheese Brunchie, Birds Eye	pack		233
Tuna Mexicana, John West	28	1	33
Walnut Gâteau Mix, Green's Microwave Magic	28	1	84

DELICATESSEN

	g	oz	Cal.
Ardennes Pâté, Mattessons	28	1	100
Black Pudding:			
average, sliced and fried	28	1	85
Mattessons	28	1	102
Bavarian Ham Sausage, St Michael	28	1	46
Bierwurst, St Michael	28	1	57
Bratwurst, Mattessons	28	1	95
Chopped Pork & Ham, Mattessons	28	1	94
Corned Beef, Fray Bentos	tinned 198	7	217

	g	oz	Cal.
Cured Pork Shoulder, St Michael	28	1	27
Cured Salt Beef, St Michael	28	1	47
Danish Salami: Chic-o-Roll	28	1	140
Sainsbury	28	1	161
Faggots, Bowyers	28	1	94
Farmers Slice, Wall's	283	10	900
Frankfurter: Mattessons	28	1	100
Sainsbury	28	1	69
French Garlic Sausage:			
Co-op	28	1	75
Sainsbury	28	1	74
Tesco	28	1	63
Garlic Sausage, Bowyers	28	1	66
German Cervelat Sausage, Sainsbury	28	1	112
German Salami, Sainsbury	28	1	120
German Style Sausage:			
Mattessons	28	1	70
Wall's	28	1	69
Ham:			
Parma, St Michael	28	1	85
honey roasted, St Michael	28	1	35
Virginia, Waitrose	28	1	46

		g	oz	Cal.
York, boiled, lean only		28	1	62
Ham Sausage, Mattessons		28	1	38
Haslet, average		28	1	80
Hickory Smoked Ham, Mattessons		28	1	24
Kabanos, Sainsbury	each			90
Liver Sausage: average		28	1	88
Bowyers		28	1	60
Lunch Tongue, Mattessons		28	1	75
Luncheon Meat: average		28	1	89
Wall's	tinned	340	12	1140
Luncheon Sausage, average		28	1	80
Parma Ham, St Michael		28	1	85
Pastrami, Mattessons		28	1	43
Pâté:				
Brussels, Mattessons		28	1	97
chicken liver with port, Mattessons		28	1	112
crab spreading, Prince's		28	1	82
liver & ham, Mattessons		28	1	85
smoked, Prince's	tinned	28	1	42
vegetable, Granose	tinned	114	4	333
Pepperami, Mattessons	stick	25	1	140

		g	oz	Cal.
Polony, Mattessons		28	1	57
Pork Breakfast Sausage, Sainsbury		28	1	77
Pork Lunch Tongue, Safeway		28	1	53
Pork Luncheon Meat:				
Armour	tinned	340	12	1040
Mattessons		28	1	54
Pork Pie, Bowyers	medium size			74
Salami:				
Belgian		28	1	130
Danish		28	1	160
Danish, Sainsbury		28	1	161
German		28	1	120
Hungarian		28	1	130
Italian, St Michael		28	1	140
Salmon Trout Fish Pâté, Faroe	pack			230
Sausage:				
Belgian liver		28	1	90
bierwurst		28	1	75
bockwurst		28	1	180
cervelat		28	1	140
chorizo		28	1	140
continental liver		28	1	80
French garlic		28	1	90
garlic		28	1	70
German Garlic, Sainsbury		28	1	90

		g	oz	Cal.
ham		28	1	50
kabanos, Roman		28	1	85
krakowska		28	1	80
mettwurst		28	1	120
mortadella		28	1	105
pastrami		28	1	65
Polish		28	1	60
polony		28	1	80
smoked		28	1	130
Sausage Roll: Bowyers		70	2	285
Bowyers, jumbo		125	4	430
Sainsbury, mini	each			100
Scotch Eggs: Bowyers	each			350
Stuffed Pork Roll, Bowyers		28	1	90
Tongue: lamb's, stewed		28	1	82
ox, boiled		28	1	83
Topside of Beef, Tesco		28	1	36
Turkey & Ham Roll, Wall's	tinned	200	7	480
Turkey Meat Loaf, Buxted		28	1	62

	g	oz	Cal.

PANCAKES, SAVOURY

	g	oz	Cal.
Chicken & Bacon, Findus	each		90
Chicken with Mushroom Crêpes, Findus	each		98
Sausage & Baked Bean, Findus	each		98
Scotch, Sainsbury	each		70
Seafood, Birds Eye	each		120
Wholemeal Mix, Quaker	28	1	105

PANCAKES, SWEET

	g	oz	Cal.
Buttermilk mix, Quaker	28	1	130
Hazelnut Pancake Mix, Quaker Mix	packet		110
Ice Cream, Daloon	each		110
Syrup & Sultana, Sunblest	each		85

PASTA AND PIZZAS

	g	oz	Cal.
Alphabetti Spaghetti with tomato sauce, Crosse & Blackwell	213	7½	127

PASTA AND PIZZAS

		g	oz	Cal.
Bolognaise, Asda Pizza			28	1	61
Cannelloni: Buitoni	tinned	400	14	380
Findus	frozen	350	12¼	435
Capricciosa Pizza, Pizza Express	each			885
Cheese Feast Pan Pizza, Pizza Hut	each			734
Cheese & Tomato Pizza, Safeway	each	180	6½	360
Four Seasons Pizza, Pizza Express	each			890
French Bread Pizza:				
Findus, Cheese & Tomato	each	142	5	333
Ross	each			300
Hawaiian Thin 'N' Crispy, Pizza Hut	each			500
Ham & Mushroom Pizza, Birds Eye	each	265	9¼	580
Ham & Pineapple Pizza, Findus	each			343
Italiana Pizza, Iceland	each			140
Lasagne:				
Birds Eye International Meal	frozen	250	8¾	375
Findus	frozen	330	11½	360
St Michael	frozen	283	10	350

		g	oz	Cal.
Long Spaghetti in sauce, Nisa	tinned	220	7¾	145
Macaroni:				
boiled		28	1	32
wholewheat, boiled, plain		28	1	32
wholewheat, raw		28	1	92
Macaroni Cheese: average		28	1	59
Iceland	packet			290
Safeway	tinned	210	7½	248
Margherita Pizza, Pizza Express	each			760
Marinara Pizza, Pizza Express	each			700
Meat Feast Pan Pizza, Pizza Hut	each			780
Mushroom Pizza, Marietta's	17.5cm(7in)			520
Mushroom Pizza, Pizza Express	each			700
Mushroom & Garlic Pizza, Iceland	each			942
Napoletana Pizza, Pizza Express	each			810
Noodles: cooked		28	1	34
raw		28	1	102
Noodle Doodles, Heinz	tinned	215	7½	135
Pepperoni Feast, Thick 'N' Thin, Pizza Hut	each			757
Pizza Base Mix, Granny Smith	packet			500

		g	oz	Cal.
Pizza Four Seasons Luxury, Birds Eye	each			600
Pizza Fingers, Marietta's	each			95
Pizza, Tomato & Cheese, Ross	12cm(5in)	28	1	62
Pot Noodles, Beef & Tomato, Golden Wonder	pot		–	335
Ravioli, Buitoni	tinned	200	7	140
Ravioli in Tomato Sauce, Heinz	tinned	215	7½	170
Seafood Fettucine, St Michael	frozen	350	12	650
Seafood Pizza, McCains		28	1	62
Spaghetti:				
boiled, plain		28	1	33
raw		28	1	107
tinned in tomato sauce		28	1	17
wholewheat, raw		28	1	97
Spaghetti Alphabet with Tomato Sauce, Crosse & Blackwell		213	7½	128
Spaghetti Hoops in Tomato Sauce, Heinz		215	7½	142
Spaghetti Rings in Tomato Sauce, Crosse & Blackwell		213	7½	134
Special Pizza, Marietta's	17cm(7in)			610

	g	oz	Cal.
Spicy Beef Curry, Golden Wonder Pot Noodles with Sauce	pot			338
Taco Shell, Old El Paso	each			50
Tagliatelli, Rossi		400	14	690
Tagliatelli & Ham, Sainsbury	packet	300	10	420
Tomato & Cheese Pizza, St Michael	each	454	16	907
Tomato & Cheese Pizza Snack:				
Birds Eye	each			270
Marietta's	12cm (5in)			210
Tortellini, Six Cheese, Pasta Co.		100	3½	176
Tortellini, Spinach & Ricotta, Sainsbury		100	3½	285
Traditional Cannelloni, McVitie's		28	1	37
Wholewheat Pasta, Record		100	3½	327
Veneziana Pizza, Pizza Express	each			750

		g	oz	Cal.

PASTRY AND BATTER

		g	oz	Cal.
Pastry:				
choux: baked		28	1	95
raw		28	1	60
flaky: baked		28	1	150
raw		28	1	115
puff: baked		28	1	115
Birds Eye		28	1	115
Jus-Rol		28	1	114
raw		28	1	115
shortcrust: baked		28	1	150
Birds Eye		28	1	125
Jus-Rol		28	1	125
Safeway		28	1	122
raw		28	1	130
wholemeal: baked		28	1	145
raw		28	1	120
Pancake Mix, Whitworth's		100	3½	348
Pastry Mix, Lyons		28	1	133
Traditional Pastry, Freshbake		149	5¼	460
Vol-au-Vent Pastry Case,				
Jus-Rol:	cocktail size			40
	medium size			72
Yorkshire Pudding: average		28	1	60
Jus-Rol	each			30
Viota mix				492

	g	oz	Cal.
Yorkshire Pudding Mix, Whitworth's	255	9	889

PIES, PIE FILLINGS, FLANS AND QUICHES
SAVOURY

		g	oz	Cal.
Bacon & Cheese Flan, Sainsbury	each			390
Beef Pie, Birds Eye Value	each			370
Cheese, Egg & Bacon Flan, Birds Eye	each			900
Cheese & Onion Quiche, St Michael		28	1	84
Chicken & Mushroom Pie:				
Fray Bentos		28	1	50
Wall's		28	1	77
Chicken & Vegetable Pie, Bowyers	each			314
Cottage Pie, Ross	each			150
Crofter Pie, Tesco		28	1	35
Family Minced Beef Pie, Asda		28	1	93

		g	oz	Cal.
Gala Pie, Bowyers		115	4	365
Meat & Potato Pie, Freshbake		113	4	350
Melton Mowbray Pie, Sainsbury	each		16	1520
Melton Mowbray Pork Pie, Wall's	each			610
Minced Beef Pie, Wall's family size	each			1090
Minced Beef & Vegetable Pie, Birds Eye	each			409
Minced Steak & Onion Pie Filling, Fray Bentos	tinned	392	15	643
Party Pork Pie, Wall's	each			1010
Pork Pie: average		28	1	104
Bowyers, individual		140	5	550
Wall's		142	5	585
Tesco, Melton Mowbray, individual		142	5	389
Potato, Leek & Cheese Flan, Sainsbury		170	6	360
Premium Pork Pie, Sainsbury		128	4½	400
Raised Pork Pie: Bowyers		530	19	1890
Wall's		454	16	1747
Salmon & Broccoli Flan, Sainsbury	each	392	14	1020

		g	oz	Cal.
Scotch Pie, Wall's		113	4	320
Shepherd's Pie, Birds Eye		227	8	275
Steak Pie, Sainsbury	each	400	5	1164
Steak & Kidney Pie: Birds Eye	each			370
Wall's		28	1	83
Steak & Kidney Pudding, Fray Bentos	tinned	213	7½	435
Steak & Mushroom Pie Filling, Fray Bentos		392	14	357
Steak & Onion Pie Filling, Fray Bentos		392	14	478
Turkey in Rich Pastry, St Michael		28	1	90
Vegetable & Steak Pie, Fray Bentos	tinned	213	7½	373
Vegetable & Steak Pie Filling, Fray Bentos	tinned	392	15	439

		g	oz	Cal.

PIES, PIE FILLINGS, FLANS AND QUICHES
SWEET

		g	oz	Cal.
Apple & Blackberry, Batchelor's Pack A Pie	jar	405	14¼	350
Apple & Blackberry Fruit Pie Filling, Mortons	tinned	385	13½	347
Apple & Raspberry, Batchelor's Pack A Pie	jar	405	14¼	350
Apple & Raspberry Fruit Pie Filling, Mortons	tinned	100	3½	88
Apricot Pie Filling, Sainsbury		397	14	357
Gooseberry Flan Filling, Armour	tin	850	30	755
Harvest Pie, Lyons:				
apple	each			355
apple & blackcurrant	each			354
Lemon Pie Filling:				
Birds Eye, made up	packet			255
Royal, made up	packet			490
Mincemeat: average		28	1	37
Hartley's		28	1	86

		g	oz	Cal.
Mince Pie: average		28	1	111
Mr Kipling	each			204
Pineapple Flan Filling, Armour	tinned	850	30	835
Plum, Batchelor's Pack A Pie		405	14¼	242
Raspberry Flan Filling, Armour	tinned	250	9	1005
Red Cherry Pie Filling, Co-op	tinned	400	14	310
Redcurrant & Raspberry, Batchelor's Pack A Pie	jar			300
Redcurrant & Raspberry Pie, Mr Kipling	each			192
Strawberry Flan Filling, Armour	tin	850	30	1105
Strawberry Fruit Pie Filling, Pickering's		395	14	312
Swiss Black Cherry Fruit Pie Filling, Sainsbury		397	14	397

POULTRY

		g	oz	Cal.
Chicken:				
breast, fried, weighed with skin & bone		175	6	215
breast, grilled, weighed with skin & bone		175	6	200

	g	oz	Cal.
drumstick, fried in egg &			
breadcrumbs, raw weight	85	3	130
meat, boiled	28	1	52
Duck:			
leg portion, baked:			
meat only	28	1	120
meat & skin	28	1	165
raw: meat only	28	1	35
meat, fat & skin	28	1	122
roast: meat only	28	1	54
meat, fat & skin	28	1	96
wing, baked: meat only	28	1	55
meat & skin	28	1	55
Goose, roast, meat only	28	1	90
Grouse, weighed with bones	28	1	32
Guinea fowl, roast & on the bone	28	1	30
Partridge: meat only	28	1	60
roast, weighed with bones	28	1	37
Pheasant: roast, weighed whole	28	1	29
roast, meat only	28	1	64
Pigeon, roast, weighed whole	28	1	29
Quail, roast, weighed whole	100	3½	90
Turkey, roast, weighed with skin & stuffing	28	1	52

		g	oz	Cal.

POULTRY DISHES

		g	oz	Cal.
Chicken Breast Far Eastern, St Michael		28	1	58
Chicken Cordon Bleu, Ross		28	1	53
Chicken in a bun, Wimpy	each			530
Chicken Kiev, St Michael	packet	312	11	820
Chicken Korma, St Michael	packet	397	14	1050
Chicken & Mushroom Casserole, Birds Eye Menu Master	packet			160
Chicken Samosa, Waitrose		28	1	52
Chicken Supreme, Beanfeast		28	1	84
Chicksticks, Birds Eye	each			65
Duck in orange sauce, average				600
Golden Chicken with Noodles, Heinz Super Mugs	tub			70
Imperial Chicken & Fried Rice, Uncle Wong		320	11½	445
Seasoned Chicken, Sage & Onion, St Michael		28	1	56
Sweet & Sour Chicken, Vesta 2-serving packet				1020

	g	oz	Cal.
Tandoori Flavour Chicken, St Michael	28	1	75

PUDDINGS

	g	oz	Cal.
Angel Delight, Bird's:			
Butterscotch, made up with semi-skimmed milk	28	1	27
Banana, made up with whole milk	28	1	33
Chocolate, made up with semi-skimmed milk	28	1	27
Wild Strawberry, made up with whole milk	28	1	33
Apple & Blackberry Crumble, Tiffany's	each		1080
Apple & Blackcurrant Pie, Lyons mini size			175
Apple Cream Dessert, St Michael	28	1	48
Apple crumble, average	28	1	57
Apple Pie: Freshbake, family size	28	1	78
Lyons, mini size	each		175

	g	oz	Cal.
Lyons, Harvest Pie			
Dessert	each		1025
McDonald's	each		229
Wimpy	each		315
Baked Alaska, Mary Baker Simply Sweet, Nabisco Frear	packet		990
Baked Jam Roll, St Michael	28	1	111
Bakewell Tart, Mr Kipling	28	1	116
Blackberry & Apple Sponge, St Michael	28	1	72
Blackcurrant Cheesecake, Waitrose	28	1	101
Blackcurrant Yoghurt Cheesecake, Homepride	serving		261
Blancmange, Brown & Polson:			
chocolate, not made up	100	4	335
vanilla, not made up	100	4	328
all other flavours not made up	100	4	328
Blueberry Muffin, Betty Crocker, prepared	100	4	340
Canary pudding, average	28	1	131
Caramel Supreme, Eden Vale	carton		158
Castle pudding, average	28	1	112

		g	oz	Cal.
Chocolate Chip Sundae, Wimpy	each			160
Chocolate Delight Dessert, St Michael		28	1	38
Chocolate Seville, Eden Vale	carton			115
Chocolate Supreme, Eden Vale	carton			170
Creamed Rice, Ambrosia	tinned	439	15½	399
Creme Caramel, Eden Vale	each			139
Custard: with cream added		28	1	56
powder		28	1	100
powder made up to 150ml(¼ pint) with skimmed milk				130
Custard tart, average		28	1	82
Dairy Custard, Co-op		425	15	500
Date Dessert, Whitworth's	tub			425
Dessert Sauces, Lyons Maid				
butterscotch		28	1	89
chocolate		28	1	81
strawberry		28	1	75
Devon Custard, Ambrosia		439	15½	440
snack size		170	6	175
Dutch Apple Tart, McVitie's		28	1	66

		g	oz	Cal.
Egg Custard Tart, St Michael	each			215
Flan Case, Lyons	each			480
Fresh Fruit Salad without cream, Pizza Express	portion			82
Fruit & Nut Sundae, Wimpy	portion			235
Fruit Cocktail Trifle, St Ivel	carton			160
Gooseberry Crumble, Tiffany's	each			1040
Instant Custard, Brown & Polson		100		403
Instant Whip, Bird's:				
chocolate	serving			590
butterscotch, toffee	serving			580
Jam roll, baked, average		28	1	115
Jam Roly Poly, Tiffany's	each			1045
Jam Tarts: average		28	1	42
Lyons	each			100
Jelly: Chivers, all flavours	block			285
	cube			30
made up with milk		28	1	25
made up with water		28	1	16
Nestlé, all flavours	block	135	4½	350
	cube			30

		g	oz	Cal.
Leicester pudding, average		28	1	192
Lemon Meringue Pie Mix, Green's, made up	packet	28	1	55
Lemon Pie Filling Mix, Green's made up	packet	28	1	26
Macaroni Pudding, Co-op	tinned	425	15	90
Mandarin & Lemon Whip, Eden Vale	carton			125
Meringue, average		28	1	110
Mince Pie: average		28	1	111
Mr Kipling		28	1	58
Mississippi Mud Pie, Young's		28	1	100
Mixed fruit pudding, average		28	1	92
Mixed Fruit Sponge, Heinz	tin	300	10½	930
Orange & Almond Pudding, McVitie's		28	1	107
Peach & Passion Fruit Shapers Dessert, Boots	sachet			125
Peach & Passion Fruit Trifle, St Michael		28	1	46
Peach Trifle, St Ivel	carton			165
Pecan Pie, Sainsbury	each			1325

		g	oz	Cal.
Pineapple Papaya Delight, Tree Free	packet	100	3½	374
Profiterole Mix, Mary Baker Nabisco Frear	packet			935
Queen of puddings, average		28	1	129
Raspberry Dessert Sauce, Wall's		28	1	31
Raspberry Jam Sponge Pudding, Heinz		75	2½	226
Raspberry Jam Sponge Pudding, Heinz		300	10½	891
Raspberry Trifle, St Ivel	carton			144
Rice Creamola, Sun-pat		225	9	910
Rice Pudding, Co-op	tinned	170	6	146
Rum Baba, McVitie's	each			205
Rum & Raisin Crunch Mix, Royal		28	1	70
Sago Pudding, Co-op	tinned	425	15	350
Semolina Pudding, Co-op	tinned	425	15	331
Spicy Apple & Sultana Pudding, Tiffany's	each			1380
Strawberry Fool, St Michael		28	1	44

		g	oz	Cal.
Strawberry Fruit Fruitfull, Beddington's	packet	142	5	180
Strawberry Jam Sponge Pudding, Heinz	tinned	300	10½	897
Strawberry Mousse, Sainsbury	carton	62.5	2¼	100
Strawberry Pavlova, McVitie's		28	1	95
Strawberry Whip, St Michael	carton			95
Tangy Lemon Cheesecake, Granny Smith Mix	packet			1520
Traditional Rice Pudding with Nutmeg and Sultanas, Ambrosia		439	15½	443
Treacle Sponge Pudding, Heinz	tinned	300	10½	903
Treacle Tart, Mr Kipling		28	1	98
Trifle Mix, Bird's, made up	packet			1280
Tropical Fruit Flan, Asda		28	1	72
Tropical Whip Dessert, St Michael		28	1	34

	g	oz	Cal.

FROZEN PUDDINGS AND ICE CREAM

	g	oz	Cal.
Apple Dessert, McVitie's cake	each		490
Apple Cream Slice, McVities's cake	each		240
Apple Pie, McVitie's	28	1	67
Apple Strudel, Asda	28	1	73
Apricot Padua, Bertorelli	28	1	50
Arctic Gâteau, Birds Eye	each		500
Arctic Roll, Birds Eye	100	3½	214
Black Cherry Ice Cream, Continental Dairy, Waitrose	28	1	53
Black Cherry Delight, Lyons Maid cutting brick	28	1	52
Blackcurrant Cheesecake, McVitie's	each		1360
Blackcurrant Sorbet, Waitrose	28	1	35
Cheesecake:			
Apple & Blackberry, Ross	28	1	65
Blackcurrant, Sainsbury	450	16	1302
Lemon & Sultana, Waitrose	28	1	92

	g	oz	Cal.
Chipwich, Lyons Maid Individual Ice Cream	each		343
Chocolate Chip Ice Cream, Lyons Maid Gold Seal	28	1	57
Chocolate Chip Ripple Ice Cream, St Michael	28	1	62
Chocolate Ice Cream, St Michael	28	1	7
Chocolate Ice Cream Gâteau, Safeway	28	1	71
Chocolate Ripple Ice Cream, Lyons Maid	brick		925
Chocolate Soft-Scoop Ice Cream, Safeway	28	1	47
Chocolate Swirl Ice Cream, Lyons Maid Gold Seal	28	1	54
Choux Buns, Birds Eye	each		120
Cointreau Gâteau, Safeway	28	1	83
Cornetto, Chocolate & Nut, Wall's	each		210
Cornetto, Magnifico, Wall's	each		320
Cornetto, Rum & Raisin, Wall's	each		195

FOOD

	g	oz	Cal.
Cornish Dairy Ice Cream, Lyons Maid	brick		903
Cornish Strawberry, King Cone, Lyons Maid	each		205
Cornish Vanilla Chocolate Ice Cream, Lyons Maid	each		126
Dairy Black Cherry Delight, Lyons Maid (Napoli)	50	2	95
Dairy Chocolate Ice Cream, Bertorelli	50	2	103
Dairy Coffee Ice Cream, Bertorelli	50	2	110
Dairy Cornish Ice Cream, Ross	50	2	90
Tesco	50	2	106
Dairy ice cream, average	50	2	130
Dairy Mela Menthe Ice Cream, Bertorelli	28	1	85
Dairy Mela Parisienne Ice Cream, Bertorelli	28	1	84
Dairy Mela Stregata Ice Cream, Bertorelli	28	1	84

	g	oz	Cal.
Dairy Nutty Toffee Ice Cream, Lyons Maid (Napoli)	50	2	110
Dairy Peach Melba Ice Cream, Lyons Maid (Napoli)	50	2	90
Dairy Praline Ice Cream, Bertorelli	50	2	130
Dairy Strawberry Ice Cream, Bertorelli	50	2	100
Dairy Strawberry Ice Cream, Lyons Maid (Napoli)	50	2	76
Dairy Tutti Fruitti Ice Cream, Lyons Maid (Napoli)	50	2	100
Dairy Vanilla Ice Cream, Bertorelli	50	2	115
Dairy Vanilla Ice Cream, Lyons Maid (Napoli)	50	2	100
Dark & Golden Choc Bar, Wall's	each		105
Dark Satin Choc Ice, Lyons Maid	each		130
Double Chocolate Cake, Birds Eye	each		930
Dracula Ice Lolly, Wall's	each		50

	g	oz	Cal.
Dream Chocolate Bar, Wall's	each		195
Eclair, Birds Eye	each		126
Freaky Foot, Wall's	each		90
Fruit & Nut Sundae, Wimpy	portion		235
Golden Orange Ice Cream, Lyons Maid	each		55
Golden Vanilla Choc Bar, Wall's	each		125
Gold Seal Caramel Toffee, Lyons Maid	28	1	57
Gold Seal Raspberry Peach Sundae, Lyons Maid	28	1	39
Gooseberry Fool, Waitrose	28	1	50
Ice Cream: average	28	1	45
Mr Whippy's	28	1	46
Ice Cream Bar, Wall's Cornish, low fat	28	1	22
Ice Cream Float, Wimpy	portion		190
Ice Cream Mix, Pearce Duff	packet		320
Ice Cream Pancakes, Daloon	each		110
Ice Cream Roll, Co-op	each		340
Ice Cream Sundae, Wimpy	portion		240

	g	oz	Cal.
Knickerbocker Glory: Iceland each			182
Wimpy portion			240
Lemon Cream Pie, Findus	28	1	103
Lemon Curd Sherbert Ice Cream, Baskin Robbins	28	1	46
Lemon Surprise, Bertorelli	28	1	32
Lemon Sorbet, Bertorelli	28	1	32
Lemon Torte, Ross	28	1	71
Light Choc Ice, Frederick's each			125
Maple Walnut Ice Cream, Hortons	28	1	57
Magnum Chocolate Bar, dark, Wall's each			290
Mela Stregata, Bertorelli	28	1	85
Midnight Mini Choc Bar, Wall's each			141
Mini Brick, Lyons Maid each			55
Mini Milk, Wall's each			35
Mini Juice Bar, Wall's each			25
Mint Choc Chip, Lyons Maid Gold Seal	28	1	59
Mint Choc Ices, Frederick's each			125
Mini Waffles, Birds Eye each			60

	g	oz	Cal.
Mint Neapolitan, Lyons Maid Soft Scoop	28	1	52
Mr Men, Lyons Maid Lollies each			27
Neapolitan Ice Cream:			
Lyons Maid cutting brick	28	1	51
Lyons Maid family brick	28	1	51
non-dairy, St Michael	28	1	50
Ross	28	1	51
soft scoop, Waitrose	28	1	45
Nobbly Bobbly, Lyons Maid each			180
Orange Fruitie Ice Lolly, Wall's each			55
Orange Maid Ice Cream, Lyons Maid each			49
Orange Maid, Lyons Maid each			50
Orange Surprise, Bertorelli portion			175
Peach Melba Ice Cream, Lyons Maid brick			920
Peach Melba Soft Scoop Bulk Ice Cream, Lyons Maid	28	1	50
Pineapple Ice Cream, Lyons Maid	28	1	43
Pineapple Juice Bar, Lyons Maid each			46

	g	oz	Cal.
Plum Pudding & Rum Sauce, Ross	each		300
Profiterole Choux, Ross	28	1	114
Raspberry Dessert Flan, Lyons Maid	28	1	75
Raspberry Ripple: Tesco	28	1	59
Ripple	brick		312
Raspberry Puffs, St Michael, frozen	28	1	108
Raspberry Supermousse, Birds Eye	carton		120
Raspberry Torte, McVitie's	28	1	77
Raspberry/Vanilla Double Mousse, Findus	tub		90
Raspberry Water Ice, Lyons Maid	28	1	22
Raspberry and Redcurrant Cheesecake, St Michael	28	1	81
Real Milk Ice, Lyons Maid	each		50
Rhum Baba, Ross	each		340
Rich Chocolate Ripple, Lyons Maid	28	1	50

	g	oz	Cal.
Roast Almond Chocolate, Lyons Maid	100	3½	545
Rock Around the Choc, Lyons Maid	each		130
Rocket Ice Cream, Lyons Maid	each		30
Rocky Road, Baskin Robbins Single Scoop Ice Cream	each		185
Rum & Raisin, Napoli Dairy, Lyons Maid	28	1	51
Skull, Lyons Maid	each		80
Strawberry & Vanilla Family Brick, Ross Tudor	50	2	110
Strawberry Creme de Creme, Lyons Maid Soft Scoop	50	2	100
Strawberry Cup Italiano, Wall's	each		115
Strawberry Mivvi, Lyons Maid	each		80
Strawberry Cheesecake, McVitie's	28	1	92
Strawberry Split, Wall's	each		80
Strawberry Sundae, Wimpy	each		140

FROZEN PUDDINGS AND ICE CREAM

		g	oz	Cal.
Supermousse, Birds Eye				
Choc & Nut	carton			150
Strawberry	carton			110
Swiss Mountain Strawberry Ice Cream, Wall's		50	2	105
Tangle Twister, Wall's	each			92
Tiramisu Gâteau, Ross	each			93
Toffee Crumble Ice Cream, Lyons Maid	each			153
Toffee Crunch Sundae, Wall's family size	each			590
Toffee Ripple, Lyons Maid, family brick	each			430
Tom & Jerry Lolly, Wall's	each			50
Totem Pole, Lyons Maid	each			80
Triple Choc Lolly, Lyons Maid	each			227
Vanilla Bar, Lyons Maid	each			70
Vanilla & Flake Milk Chocolate, Loseley		28	1	44
Vanilla Ice Cream:				
Baskin Robbins		70	2½	142
Horton's		28	1	49
Tesco Easy Scoop		28	1	53

		g	oz	Cal.
Vanilla Ripple, Co-op		28	I	41
Viennetta Capuccino, Wall's Special		28	I	37
Water ice, average		28	I	20
Woppa, Wall's	each			40
Yoghurt, iced, Sainsbury		28	I	118
Zoom, Lyons Maid	each			38

RICE AND RICE DISHES

		g	oz	Cal.
Chicken Curry: Batchelor's Vesta Meal	portion			392
Golden Wonder	pot			240
Chicken Savoury Rice, Batchelor's	packet	120	4¼	406
Golden Rice, Batchelor's	packet	120	4¼	408
Mild Curry, Batchelor's Savoury Rice	packet	120	4¼	393
Mixed Vegetable Savoury, Gateway		28	I	33

		g	oz	Cal.
Paella, Vesta	each helping			325
Pilau Rice, Olaf Foods	packet			234
Pot Rice, Chicken Supreme, Golden Wonder	packet			245
Rice:				
basmati, raw		28	1	102
brown: boiled		28	1	30
raw		28	1	100
white: boiled		28	1	35
raw		28	1	102
Rice, Peas & Mushrooms, Birds Eye	packet	227	8	318
Risotto, KP	tub			150
Sweet & Sour Savoury Rice, Batchelor's	packet	121		419
Savoury Spanish Rice, Safeway, Boil in the Bag	packet			92
Yang Chow Fried Rice	pack	170	6	305

SALADS

		g	oz	Cal.
American, Asda		28	1	47

	g	oz	Cal.
Apple, peach & nut, average	28	1	58
Celery, Apple & Orange, Mattessons	28	1	55
Chicken & Sweetcorn, Eden Vale	28	1	44
Classic Coleslaw, Eden Vale	28	1	87
Crispy, in Vinaigrette, St Ivel	28	1	20
Crunchy Coleslaw, Eden Vale	28	1	88
Egg, Cheese and Chives Potato with salad filling, Spud-U-Like each			335
Florida, St Michael	227	8	465
French in Vinaigrette, Mattessons	227	8	185
Malaysian, Eden Vale	160	5½	428
Pasta: Eden Vale serving			431
Heinz tinned	210	17½	400
St Michael	227	8	400
Potato & Chive: Eden Vale	227	8	368
Sainsbury	28	1	57
Potato & Frankfurter, St Ivel	28	1	40
Prawn, average	142	5	150
Prawn coleslaw, average	200	7	215

		g	oz	Cal.
Spanish, Eden Vale		28	1	30
Spicy Potato, Safeway		28	1	56
Spicy Rice, Eden Vale		170	6	350
Spring, Mattessons		170	6	300
Three Bean Salad, St Michael Pot Salad		28	1	39
Tzatziki, Sainsbury		28	1	29
Vegetable: Eden Vale	carton	227	8	390
Safeway		28	1	59
Waldorf, Tesco		50	2	107
Wild Rice, Waitrose		28	1	47

SAUCES, STUFFINGS AND DRESSINGS
SAVOURY

		g	oz	Cal.
Au Poivre Sauce, Crosse & Blackwell	sachet	100	3½	357
Barbecue Dry Sauce Mix, Colman's		28	1	41

	g	oz	Cal.
Beef Bourguignon, Colman's Casserole Mix	28	1	99
Beef Goulash, Cook-in-the-Pot, Crosse & Blackwell	28	1	93
Beef Provençale, Cook-in-the-Pot, Crosse & Blackwell	28	1	93
Beef Stroganoff, Cook-in-the-Pot, Crosse & Blackwell	28	1	97
Blue Cheese Dressing:			
Kraft	28	1	135
Sainsbury	28	1	147
Bolognese Sauce:			
Buitoni	100	4	60
Sainsbury	28	1	44
Bread Sauce:			
fresh, average	1 tablespoon		15
Colman's Dry Mix	28	1	94
Brown Sauce, Gateway	28	1	40
Chicken Chasseur, Cook-in-the-Pot, Crosse & Blackwell	28	1	97
Chicken Seasoning, Colman's Dry Sauce Mix	28	1	90
Chilli Sauce, HP	28	1	35
Original French Dressing, Kraft	28	1	139

	g	oz	Cal.
Cook-in-Sauce, Homepride:			
French Red Wine	28	1	28
Indian Curry	28	1	18
Texas Barbecue	28	1	19
Curry dressing, average	28	1	42
Curry Casserole Sauce, Knorr	28	1	26
Daddies Burger Relish	28	1	25
Daddies Tomato Ketchup, HP	28	1	33
Daddies Tomato Sauce, HP	28	1	20
Dopiaza Curry Sauce, Homepride	28	1	26
Egg mayonnaise, average helping			260
English Herb Dressing, Alfonal	28	1	100
Fletchers Tiger Sauce, HP	28	1	32
French dressing: average	1 tablespoon		75
oil free	1 tablespoon		3
Fruity Sauce, HP	28	1	33
Garlic & Herbs Stuffing Mix, Knorr	100		410
Garlic Salad Dressing, St Michael	28	1	185

	g	oz	Cal.
Gravy:			
Lite, McCormicks Gravy Mix, made up 3 tablespoons			9
powder, Bisto	3	1/16	8
thick, average, made with dripping 2 tablespoons			30
Hazelnut & Herb Stuffing Mix:			
average	28	1	121
Knorr	100		428
Hot Taco Sauce, Old El Paso	28	1	10
HP Mint Sauce	28	1	44
HP Sauce	28	1	28
Italian Garlic Dressing, Kraft	28	1	119
Korma Authentic Curry Sauce, Sharwood tin	283	10	249
Korma Classic Curry Sauce, Homepride tin	380	13½	590
Korma Curry Mix, Colman's packet			145
Lamb Ragoût, Cook-in-the-Pot, Crosse & Blackwell	28	1	97
Madeira Wine Gravy, Crosse & Blackwell	100	4	358
Madras Curry, Asda	28	1	96

		g	oz	Cal.
Madras Curry Sauce, Homepride	tinned	383	13½	401
Mayonnaise: average		28	1	205
Hellmann's		28	1	201
Tesco		28	1	200
Mexican dressing, Safeway		28	1	172
Mild Taco Sauce, Old El Paso		28	1	10
Mint Jelly:				
Colman's		28	1	75
Frank Cooper		28	1	78
Mint sauce, average	1 teaspoon			5
Mushroom Gravy Mix, McCormick		28	1	9
Mushrooom Ketchup, Burgess		28	1	8
Mushroom Sauce Mix, Colman's		28	1	104
Mustard Vinaigrette, Tesco		28	1	129
Napolitan Sauce: Asda	tinned	28	1	13
Campbells	tinned	28	1	26
OK Fruity Sauce, Colman's		28	1	26
Onion Dry Sauce Mix, Colman's		28	1	90
Onion Sauce, Knorr Pour Over		28	1	20
Onion sauce, average		28	1	25

FOOD

		g	oz	Cal.
Onion Sauce Mix: Colman's	packet			90
Safeway	sachet			106
Parsley & Chives Salad Dressing, Knorr	sachet			20
Parsley Sauce: Colman's Mix	packet			100
Knorr Mix		100	4	348
Parsley & Thyme Stuffing:				
Paxo mix	packet			292
Whitworth's mix	packet	85	3	300
Pizzaiola Sauce, St Michael		28	1	16
Pork, Colman's Casserole Mix		28	1	84
Prawn Cocktail Sauce, Burgess		28	1	103
Red Wine Sauce, Knorr Casserole Recipe	tinned	28	1	23
Rogan Josh Curry Sauce, Homepride	tinned	383	13½	314
Sage & Onion Stuffing: Knorr		100	3½	404
Paxo	packet			300
Salad Cream, Crosse & Blackwell		100	3½	370
Sauce Tartare, Burgess		28	1	82
Seafood Dressing, Pearce & Duff		28	1	139

		g	oz	Cal.
Sunflower Dressing, Flora	1 tablespoon			75
Sweet & Sour Sauce, HP		28	1	40
Tandoori Marinade Curry Mix, Colman's	packet			92
Tandoori Sauce, HP		28	1	29
Tartare Sauce: average		28	1	82
Frank Cooper		28	1	88
Pearce Duff		28	1	82
Sharwood		28	1	80
Thousand Island Dressing:				
Hellman's fat free		28	1	118
Kraft		28	1	110
Safeway		28	1	77
Thousand Island Reduced Calorie, Kraft		28	1	50
Tomato Ketchup:				
average		28	1	28
Crosse & Blackwell		28	1	35
HP		28	1	28
Tomato & Onion Cook in Sauce, Homepride	tin	376	13½	260
Tomato Classic Italian Ketchup, Sainsbury				32
Vinaigrette, Eden Vale		28	1	9

		g	oz	Cal.
Vindaloo Authentic Curry Sauce, Sharwood	tinned	28	1	25
Virginia Bell Pepper Sauce, Schwartz	packet			120
White sauce, savoury, average		28	1	41
White Wine Sauce, Crosse & Blackwell	sachet	100	3½	365
Worcestershire Sauce, Lea & Perrins		28	1	20
Yogurt & Chive Dressing, Heinz		28	1	83
Yogurt & Cucumber Dressing, Burgess		28	1	93

SAUCES, STUFFINGS AND DRESSINGS
SWEET

	g	oz	Cal.
Bramley Apple Sauce, Pan-Yan	28	1	16
Brandy butter, average	28	1	170
Butterscotch Sauce, Lyons Maid	28	1	90

		g	oz	Cal.
Caramel Topping, Colman's		28	1	85
Cranberry Jelly:				
average		28	1	40
jellied, Baxter's		28	1	71
Dream Topping, Bird's	packet	36		244
Golden syrup, average	1 tablespoon			60
Maple syrup, average		28	1	68
Profiteroles Sauce, frozen, Ross		28	1	96
Redcurrant Sauce, John West	tinned	99	3½	210
Treacle, black, average		28	1	72
Whip Topping, Rich's	30ml/1 fl oz			20
White sauce, sweet, average		28	1	47

SAVOURY SNACKS AND CRISPS

		g	oz	Cal.
Bacon Crispies, Sainsbury	packet	50	1¾	250
Bacon Crisps, KP	packet	26		135
Bacon Fries, Smiths	packet			137
Bacon Puffs, Tesco	packet	50	1¾	245

		g	oz	Cal.
Bacon Streaks, Safeway	packet	50	1¾	240
Barbecue Rings, St Michael		28	1	149
Brontosaurus Ribs, Sainsbury	packet	25	1	120
Butterkist Popcorn		28	1	111
Californian Corn Chips, Phileas Fogg	packet	40	1½	230
Cheese & Celery Sticks Biscuit, Huntley & Palmer	each			22
Cheeselets, Peak Frean	each			5
Cheese Buttons, Tesco	packet	25	1	115
Cheese & Onion Crisps, Tesco	packet	25	1	133
Cheese Sandwich Biscuits, Waitrose		28	1	141
Cheese Savouries, Gateway		28	1	150
Cheesy Corn Curls, Gateway		28	1	128
Cheese & Onion Flavour Savouries Biscuit, Limmits Meal Replacement	each meal			210
Cheese Flavour Cracker Biscuit with Bran, Limmits Meal Replacement Biscuit	each meal			210

		g	oz	Cal.
Crinkles, St Michael	packet	100	3½	530
Crunch 'n' Slim Biscuit, Crunch 'n' Slim (2 biscuits)	each meal			234
Disco: all flavours, KP	packet	30		147
ready salted, KP	packet	30		148
Frazzles, Smiths	smallest packet	26	1	120
Garlic Mini Breads, Safeway		28		150
Good 'n' Crunchy Crisps, Salt & Vinegar, KP		26	1¼	135
Hula Hoops KP:				
salt & barbecue	packet	30	1	155
salt & vinegar	packet	30	1	155
Loops, savoury snack, St Michael		28	1	136
Minced Beef Savoury Toast, warmed, Findus	each			140
Monster Munch, Smiths	packet	26	1	147
Mumbo Jumbos, all flavours, Holly Mills	packet	20	¾	87
Onion Rings, Co-op		28	1	148
Peanut Butter Wheateats, Allinson		28	1	139

		g	oz	Cal.
Peanut & Sesame Cookies, Holly Mills	each			54
Piccolos, savoury snack, Sainsbury	packet	50	2	245
Pizza Cracker Biscuit, Sainsbury	each			15
Popcorn, average		28	1	137
Pork scratchings, average		28	1	185
Potato Rings: St Michael	packet	75	2½	403
Sainsbury	packet	28	1	141
Tesco	packet	25		130
Potato Squares, Sainsbury	packet	50	2	230
Potato Swirls with Garlic Dip, Sainsbury		100	3½	483
Potato Waffles, St Michael		50	1¾	236
Prawn Cocktail Snacks, Tesco		16	½	82
Prawn Cocktail Skips, KP		18	¾	93
Punjabi Puri, Phileas Fogg	packet	40	1½	225
Quavers, Smiths	packet	18	½	93
Ready Salted Crisps, KP	packet	26	1	135
Ringos, all flavours, Golden Wonder	packet	21	¾	97

		g	oz	Cal.
Samosa Roll, Chic-o-Roll	each			165
Salt & Vinegar Crisps, St Michael		28	1	150
Savoury Puffs, Waitrose	packet	50	1¾	282
Savoury Twigs, Safeway	packet	50	1¾	196
Scampi Fries, Smiths	smallest packet			115
Sesame Cracker, Waitrose		28		138
Skips, KP		18	½	92
Snaps, Walkers	packet	14	½	75
Space Raiders, Cheese, KP	packet	18	½	85
Square Crisps, Smiths	smallest packet	25	1	135
Toasty Grills, Danish Prime	each			300
Tortilla Chips, Tesco		25	1	126
Tubes, Smiths:				
Cheese & Onion	packet			95
Salt & Vinegar	packet			95
TUC, Savoury Sandwich Biscuit, McVitie's	each			78
Turkey Savouries, Tiffany's		92		175
Twiglets, Peak Frean	long, each			5
Twists, Smiths	packet			85

		g	oz	Cal.
Wholemeal Toasties, Granose	packet	200	7½	300
Wotsits, Cheesey, Golden Wonder	packet	23	¾	115
Worcester Sauce Crisps, KP		26	¾	135

SIMPLY FOR SLIMMERS

		g	oz	Cal.
Beeflike Flavour, Soyapro Protein Food		28	1	59
Boldo Tablet, Potter's Herbal Supplies	each			18
Cambridge Diet Meal Bar, Chocolate Flavour	bar	52	1¾	140
Cambridge Diet Meal, Chicken Flavour Soup Mix	sachet	34		110
Canderel, sweetener	tablet			9
Cheese & Onion Flavour Savouries, Limmits Meal Replacement Biscuit	meal			210
Cheese Flavour Cracker Biscuit with Bran, Limmits Meal Replacement Biscuit	meal			210

	g	oz	Cal.
Chocolate Digestive Biscuit Meal, Limmits Meal Replacement Biscuit	meal		206
Crunch 'n' Slim Biscuit, Chocolate & Raisin Crunch 'n' Slim (2 biscuits)	meal		220
Dietdays, Healthcrafts Meal Replacement Biscuit	28	1	125
Diet 25 Coleslaw Salad, Eden Vale	28	1	17
Fibretrim, Healthcrafts Meal Replacement Biscuit	28	1	14
Figure Trim, Health & Diet Food Co	capsule		8
Five Day Place Replacement, Healthcrafts	28	1	101
Formula 3+6, Health & Diet Food Co	capsule		8
Fortify Meal Replacement	sachet	44	1½	200
Fruit & Nut, Meal Replacement Chocolate Bar, Boots	each		340
Glucose, liquid, BP	28	1	90
Granulated Sweetener, Sugaree	28	1	102

	g	oz	Cal.
Healthy Balance Tomato Ketchup, Crosse & Blackwell	28	1	26
Lasagne Verde, Findus Lean Cuisine	portion		241
Lessen, Slimmers' Product	meal		148
Low Calorie Coleslaw, Eden Vale	160	5½	98
Low Calorie Dressing, Heidelberg	28	1	16
Low Calorie Salad Dressing, Burgess	28	1	35
Low Calorie Tomato Ketchup, Heinz Weight Watchers	28	1	15
Low Calorie Vinaigrette, Kraft	28	1	30
Low fat spread, average	28	1	5
Low Fat Natural 1, Speise Quark Soft Cheese, Nordmilch	28	1	158
Low Fat Soft Cheese, Safeway	28	1	26
Low Fat Soft Cheese with Apricots, Senoble	28	1	40
Low Fat Spread: Outline	28	1	105

	g	oz	Cal.
Heinz Weight Watchers	28	1	100
Low Sugar Jam, Energen	28	1	36
Macaroni Provençale, Boots Snack Pot	each		154
Mayonnaise, Heinz Weight Watchers	28	1	86
Milk Chocolate Sweetmeal with Bran, Limmits Meal Replacement Biscuit	meal		206
Minced Soya & Onion Mix, Direct Foods	28	1	100
Mixed Fruit Chocolate Lunch Bar, Limmits Meal	meal		210
Muesli: with Bran, Limmits	meal		210
sugar free, Sunpure	28	1	96
Sugarfree, Holly Mills	28	1	102
Natural Protoveg, Direct Foods	28	1	80
Nut & Raisin Carob Bar, no sugar, Kalibu	each	42	1½	208
Oil, Limmits Spray & Fry	28	1	220
Orange Flavour with Bran, Limmits Replacement Meal Biscuit	meal		210

		g	oz	Cal.
Orange Marmalade, Country Basket, sugar-free jam		28	1	35
Outline Low Fat Spread		28	1	105
Oxtail Soup:				
Co-op	tinned	425	15	180
Waistline, low calorie		283	10	65
Pasta Shells, Heinz Weight Watchers	portion			225
Pepperoni Pizza, Heinz Weight Watchers	each			244
Pineapple Dance Complete Shaping Slim Plan, Weider	each			200
Prawn Curry with Rice, Findus Lean Cuisine	portion			280
Protose, Granose	tinned	248	10	455
Prune Yogurt, Waistline		125	4½	71
Reduced Calorie French Mayonnaise, Sainsbury		28	1	77
Shape Milk, St Ivel	568ml/1 pint			255
Shapers Low Calorie Dressing, Boots	1 tablespoon			25
Shapers Lunch bars, Boots:				
Orange Citrus	each			207

	g	oz	Cal.
Spicy Apple each			195
Tangy Apricot each			207
White Chocolate Coated each			224
Slender Bar, Date & Peanut, Carnation Meal Replacement each			132
Slender Plan Crunchy Muesli Carnation Meal Replacement made with whole milk sachet			318
Slender Yoghurt Enriched, Carnation Replacement Meal sachet			108
Slim Bran Biscuit, Blakey's each			35
Slim Choc, Carnation sachet			38
Slimgard Liquid Meal Replacement, strawberry, Slimgard meal			325
Slim Soup, Carnation sachet			40
Slimway Low Calorie Salad Dressing, Heinz 1 tablespoon			25
Slimmer's sugar, Sucron	28	1	108
Slymbar, Holly Mills each			115
Slymbred, Blakey's: brown slice			10
white slice			10

	g	oz	Cal.
Slymsnack, Blakey's	each			90
Slymsquare Biscuit, Blakey's	each			30
Soup:			
Tomato: Boots Shaper Soup	packet			32
Heinz low calorie	tinned	295	10½	77
Knorr, low calorie		100	3½	274
Turkey Broth, Boots Shaper Soup	packet	290	10¼	47
Vegetable: Boots Shaper Soup	packet			40
Heinz low calorie	tin	295	10½	68
Sprinkle Sweet, Hermesetas		28	1	100
Strawberry Yogurt, Waistline	carton	125	4½	75
Sugar Free Drinking Chocolate, Carnation				
made up with skimmed milk	packet			330
made up with whole milk	packet			435
Sweet 'n' Slim, Slimcea		28	1	108
Sweetener, Sweetex Powder		28	1	100
Turkey Supreme, Olida	portion			220
Vanilla Flavour with Bran, Limmits Replacement Biscuit	meal			250
Vegetable Risotto, Heinz Weight Watchers	portion			270

	g	oz	Cal.
Vita Fiber, Bayer Tablet	28	1	51
Waistline Oil-free French Dressing, Crosse & Blackwell	28	1	3
Waistline Seafood Sauce, Crosse & Blackwell	28	1	40
Weight Watchers Ice Cream Brick, Lyons Maid	brick		527
Weiners, Granose	tin 385	13½	811
Whole Earth No Sugar Ketchup, Harmony	28	1	28
Yogurt:			
diet strawberry, Ski	125	4½	50
low fat, rhubarb, Sainsbury	150	5¼	140

SOUPS

	g	oz	Cal.
Asparagus: Hugli Instant	28	1	100
Knorr Quick	sachet		48
Beef & Tomato, Batchelor's Slim-a-Soup	56	2	56
Beef Consommé, Baxter's	28	1	13
Boston Bean, Knorr	packet 28	1	270

	g	oz	Cal.
Chicken & Leek, Batchelor's Cup-a-Soup	sachet		80
Chicken & Mushroom, Batchelor's Snack-a-Soup	sachet		190
Chicken Noodle, Knorr	100		335
Chicken & Vegetable Broth with Rice, Campbells Granny	28	1	13
Cock-a-Leekie, Baxter's	28	1	6
Country Vegetable, Heinz Condensed	tinned		9
Cream of Asparagus, Baxter's	tinned	425	15	280
Cream of Celery, Heinz	28	1	12
Cream of Chicken, Campbells Condensed	tinned		28
Cream of Mushroom, Crosse & Blackwell	28	1	15
Cream of Pheasant, Baxter's	tinned	100	3½	60
Cream of Scampi, Baxter's	tinned	100	3½	54
Crofters Thick Vegetable, Knorr	packet	100	3½	280
Cullen Skink, Baxter's	100	3½	85

SOUPS

		g	oz	Cal.
Five Vegetables & Beef, Crosse & Blackwell	tinned	100	3½	40
Gazpacho, Waitrose	tinned	28	1	12
Golden Chicken & Mushroom, Heinz	tinned	300	10½	129
Golden Pea with Ham, Campbells Granny Soup	tinned	425	15	250
Golden Vegetable:				
Batchelor's Slim-a-Soup	sachet			60
Batchelor's Cup-a-Soup	sachet			75
Tesco	sachet			50
Harvest Vegetable & Chicken, Batchelor's		28	1	62
Ham, Turkey & Vegetable, Campbells Main Course		28	1	17
Highlander's Broth, Baxter's Tartan Range	tinned	100	3½	45
Highland Lentil, Knorr	packet			301
Highland Scotch Broth, Knorr	packet	100		318
Italian Tomato & Vegetable, Batchelor's made up	sachet			100
Lentil, Campbells	tinned	300	10½	273
Lentil & Bacon, Co-op	tinned	300	10½	114

		g	oz	Cal.
Lobster Bisque:				
Baxter's		425	15	229
Crosse & Blackwell Bonne				
Cuisine Soup	sachet	28	1	112
Sainsbury	jar	100	3½	35
Malaysian Chicken &				
Sweetcorn, Knorr	sachet			214
Minestrone:				
Batchelor's Cup-a-Soup	575ml/1 pint			
	packet			79
Knorr Special Recipe Quick	packet			46
Sainsbury	575ml/1 pint			
	sachet			80
Mulligatawny Spicy, Heinz	tinned	217	8	125
Mushroom, Cream of:				
Batchelor's Cup-a-Soup	sachet			96
Safeway	packet			108
Onion, Cream of, Batchelor's				
Cup-a-Soup	sachet			110
Oxtail:				
Batchelor's Cup-a-Soup				77
Campbells Bumper Harvest	tinned	392	14	153
Crosse & Blackwell Box Soup		28	1	10
Heinz	tinned	300	10½	132
Safeway	tinned	425	15	153

		g	oz	Cal.
Sainsbury	575ml/1 pint			
	tinned	283		145
Supermug	tub			85
Tesco	tinned	425	15	157
Pea & Ham:				
Baxter's	tinned	425	15	319
Campbells Main Course	tinned	425	15	360
Heinz	tinned	300	10½	162
Knorr Mix		100	3½	323
Safeway	tinned	28	1	17
Potato & Leek, Batchelor's				
Cup-a-Soup	sachet			110
Rich Tomato, Crosse &				
Blackwell Box Soup		28	1	94
Royal Game, Baxter's	tinned	425	15	136
Scotch Broth, Batchelor's				
made up	packet			273
Scottish Lentil with Vegetable,				
Crosse & Blackwell		283	10	125
Spring Vegetable, Crosse &				
Blackwell, made up		28	1	76
Stockpot, Campbells				
Condensed	tin	140	5	80
Thick Chicken:				
Crosse & Blackwell Box Soup		28	1	108
Safeway	tin	425	15	130

		g	oz	Cal.
Thick Country Vegetable, Crosse & Blackwell	packet	28	1	109
Thick Devon Onion, Batchelor's	packet			174
Thick Farmhouse Vegetable, Batchelor's	packet			132
Thick Vegetable, Gateway	sachet			135
Thick Onion, Crosse & Blackwell	packet	28	1	97
Tomato:				
Batchelor's Cup-a-Soup	sachet			78
Campbells Condensed	tin	140	5	90
Sainsbury	tin	425	15	290
Tomato with Prawns, Frank Cooper	tin	425	15	174
Tomato & Vegetable, Crosse & Blackwell Chunky	tin	432	15½	220
Traditional Vegetable & Beef, Batchelor's	packet			179
Tuna & Sweetcorn, Prewetts	tinned	425	15	190
Turkey, Frank Cooper	tinned	425	15	212
Turkey & Vegetable Broth, Campbells Condensed	tinned	140	5	100

		g	oz	Cal.
Tuscan Bean	tinned	28	1	5
Vegetable:				
Heinz	tinned	28	1	11
Tesco	tinned	425	15	168
Waitrose	tinned	28	1	13
Vegetable & Beef:				
Gateway	sachet			140
Tesco	packet			78
Vichyssoise:				
Crosse & Blackwell	tinned	425	15	229
Prewetts	packet			215
Watercress, Sainsbury	jar	28	1	10

SPREADS AND TOPPINGS

		g	oz	Cal.
Anchovy Paste, Shippams		28	1	53
Beef Paste, Prince's	jar			161
Cheese, Heinz Weight Watchers		28	1	50
Cheese Spread Triangle, Kerrygold		28	1	75
Chicken Paste, Tesco		28	1	65

		g	oz	Cal.
Crab Paste, Safeway		28	1	53
Cucumber Spread, Heinz		28	1	52
Dairy Cheese Spread:				
Nestlé		28	1	75
Sun-Pat		28	1	75
Dairylea Cheese Spread, Kraft		28	1	52
	box			280
Fish paste, average		28	1	47
Gold Dairy Spread, St Ivel		28	1	85
Golden syrup, average	1 tablespoon			60
Ham & Cheese Toast Topper, Heinz		28	1	30
Ham Spread, Prince's		28	1	65
Ham & Mustard Paste, Shippams		35	1¼	70
Honey, average		28	1	90
Honey Bear Spread, Bear Brand		28	1	82
Light Philadelphia & Salmon Spread, Kraft		28	1	54
Liver & Bacon Paste, Shippams		35	1¼	67
Malt extract, average		28	1	86

		g	oz	Cal.
Marmite		28	1	2
Meat paste, average		28	1	61
Melbury Cheese Spread, Dairy Crest		28	1	89
Mushroom & Bacon Toast Topper, Heinz	tinned	130	4½	113
Peanut Butter: average		28	1	180
Co-op		28	1	172
Gales Crunchy		28	1	170
Sun-Pat		28	1	177
Pear & Apple Spread, Harmony		28	1	73
Philadelphia, Kraft		28	1	89
Pilchard & Tomato Paste, Shippams		28	1	44
Plain Cheese Half Fat Spread, Delight		28	1	54
Potted Salmon with Butter, St Michael		28	1	47
Salmon & Shrimp, Shippams		28	1	55
Sandwich Spread, Heinz		28	1	58
Sardine & Tomato Spread, Sainsbury		53	1¾	95
Smokey Bacon Spread, Prince's		53	1¾	110

	g	oz	Cal.
Tastex Spread, Granose	28	1	60
Tuna & Mayonnaise Spread, Sainsbury	53	1¾	140
Vegetable Pâté Wholemeal Toastie, Granose	28	1	85
Whip Topping, Rich's 30ml/1 fl oz			20

VEGETABLES

	g	oz	Cal.
Ackee	28	1	43
Artichoke, boiled	28	1	3
Asparagus, boiled	28	1	3
Aubergine, uncooked	28	1	4
Avocado pear, weighed without stone	28	1	26
Baked beans:			
Chef, with hamburgers	28	1	30
Crosse & Blackwell, in tomato sauce	28	1	21
Heinz, in tomato sauce	28	1	21
Spar	28	1	24
with pork sausages, average	28	1	35

		g	oz	Cal.
Bamboo shoots, average	tinned	28	1	5
Beans:				
aduki: boiled		28	1	94
raw weight		28	1	94
baked, average	tinned	28	1	20
black eye: boiled		28	1	38
raw		28	1	93
broad: boiled		28	1	14
raw		28	1	10
buttered: boiled		28	1	77
raw		28	1	77
cannellini, average	tinned	28	1	25
French, boiled		28	1	10
flageolet, boiled		28	1	32
haricot: boiled		28	1	26
raw		28	1	77
lima, raw, dry weight		28	1	92
mung, raw, dry weight		28	1	92
red kidney: average	tinned	28	1	25
raw, dry weight		28	1	77
runner: boiled		28	1	5
raw		28	1	7
snap, raw, green		28	1	10
soya: boiled		28	1	50
raw, dry weight		28	1	108
Beetroot: boiled		28	1	12
raw		28	1	8

	g	oz	Cal.
Beetroot in Vinaigrette, St Michael	28	1	47
Broad Beans, Birds Eye	28	1	17
Broccoli: boiled	28	1	5
raw	28	1	1
Broccoli Spears, frozen, Findus	28	1	8
Broccoli Stir Fry, St Michael	28	1	8
Brussels sprouts: boiled	28	1	5
frozen, Ross	28	1	10
raw	28	1	7
Butter beans: Batchelor's	223	7¾	151
Tesco	28	1	20
Cabbage			
boiled	28	1	4
raw	28	1	6
red, pickled, average	28	1	3
red, raw	28	1	6
Savoy, boiled	28	1	3
spring, boiled	28	1	2
Carrots: boiled	28	1	5
raw	28	1	6
Smedley's tinned	28	1	19
Cassava, fresh	28	1	43

	g	oz	Cal.
Cauliflower:			
boiled	28	1	3
florets, frozen, Ross	28	1	5
raw	28	1	4
Cauliflower Stir-fry, frozen, St Michael	28	1	13
Celeriac: boiled	28	1	4
raw	28	1	8
Celery: boiled	28	1	1
braised	28	1	2
raw	28	1	2
Chick peas: boiled	28	1	42
raw	28	1	91
Chicory, raw	28	1	3
Chinese leaves, boiled	28	1	2
Chinese Vegetables, Iceland, mixed	28	1	35
Country Vegetables, frozen, Findus	28	1	16
Cucumber, raw	28	1	3
Curried Beans with Sultanas, Heinz	28	1	33
Endive	28	1	3

		g	oz	Cal.
Garden Peas, Morton's	tinned	300	10½	141
Garlic				0
Green Beans, Green Giant		28	1	12
Gherkins, pickled, Epicure		28	1	5
Haricots Verts, frozen, Findus		28	1	19
Horseradish, raw		28	1	17
Italian Beans, Heinz		28	1	27
Leek, raw		28	1	9
Lentils: brown, boiled		28	1	32
brown, uncooked		28	1	104
Lettuce		28	1	3
Marrow: boiled		28	1	2
raw		28	1	5
Mexicorn, Green Giant		28	1	20
Mint, fresh		28	1	3
Mixed Chinese Vegetables, Hartley's	tinned	38	1¼	175
Mung Beans, Tesco		28	1	35
Mushrooms: fried in butter		28	1	62
raw		28	1	2
Mushrooms in Brine, Chesswood		213	7½	15

		g	oz	Cal.
Mushy Peas: Batchelor's	tinned	300	10½	252
Morton's		300	10½	225
Mustard & Cress		28	1	3
New Potatoes, Prince's	tinned	28	1	15
Okra, raw		28	1	5
Onion:				
boiled		28	1	4
cocktail	each			1
fried		28	1	98
pickled: average	each			5
Epicure		28	1	4
Sweet, Epicure		28	1	7
raw		28	1	7
rings: in batter, fried, average		28	1	75
Ross		28	1	68
Safeway	packet	50	1¾	260
Sainsbury	packet	50	1¾	143
spring	each			3
Original Mixed Vegetables, Birds Eye		28	1	13
Oven Chips, Safeway		28	1	36
Parsley, fresh		28	1	6
Parsnip: boiled		28	1	15
roasted		28	1	30

		g	oz	Cal.
Peas:				
dried: boiled		28	1	29
raw		28	1	81
fresh: boiled		28	1	14
raw		28	1	18
mange tout: boiled		28	1	12
raw		28	1	16
split: dried and boiled		28	1	33
dried, raw		28	1	87
tinned: garden		28	1	13
processed		28	1	23
processed, Morton's		28	1	22
Peas & Baby Carrots, frozen, Birds Eye		28	1	17
Peas & Carrots, Smedley's	tinned	425	15	165
Pepper:				
green, purple, red or yellow		28	1	4
Whitworth's, dried		28	1	60
Petits Pois à la Française, St Michael		28	1	20
Petit Pois, Tesco	tinned	397	14	163
Pinto Beans, Tesco		28	1	38
Pimento, tinned in brine, average		28	1	6

		g	oz	Cal.
Plantain: green, boiled		28	1	35
green, raw		28	1	32
ripe, fried in butter		28	1	75
Potato:				
baked, whole		28	1	23
boiled, new		28	1	21
chips: Safeway, frozen		28	1	40
Tesco, frozen crinkle		28	1	71
Wimpy	portion			250
Croquettes, Findus, frozen		28	1	26
Grill, Findus		28	1	40
New, Gateway	tinned	28	1	18
Noisettes, Ross	each			52
Oven Crunches, Ross		28	1	53
Pommes Noisettes, Jus-Rol	each			10
Sauté, Findus		28	1	36
Scoops, Gateway		28	1	170
sweet: boiled		28	1	24
raw		28	1	26
Radish	each			2
Red Kidney Beans, Prince's	tinned	28	1	25
Salsify, boiled		28	1	5
Saveloy, raw	each			230
Sea kale, boiled		28	1	2

	g	oz	Cal.
Southern Vegetables, Safeway			
Stirfry	28	1	16
Spinach: boiled	28	1	9
Findus, creamed,			
frozen	28	1	18
leaf, Morton's	28	1	6
raw	28	1	7
Spring greens	28	1	3
Spring onions, raw	28	1	10
Stirfry Baby Sweetcorn,			
Sainsbury	28	1	18
Stir Fry Vegetables with Sweet			
& Sour Sauce, St Michael	340	12	310
Surprise Peas, Batchelor's	62		119
Swedes: boiled	28	1	5
diced, Waitrose	28	1	7
raw	28	1	6
Sweetcorn: cob, medium size			155
frozen, average	28	1	25
in brine tinned	28	1	22
Sweetcorn Niblets,			
Green Giant	28	1	20
Tomato: fried	28	1	19
raw	28	1	6

	g	oz	Cal.
Turnips: boiled	28	1	4
raw	28	1	6
Water Chestnuts, Sharwood	28	1	15
Watercress	28	1	4
Whole Asparagus Spears, Green Giant	28	1	5
Yams, boiled	28	1	32
Yellow Split Peas, Whitworth's	28	1	25

VEGETARIAN DISHES

Cauliflower Cheese, St Michael		28	1	30
Celeriac Florentine, Froqual	portion			250
Cheese & Onion Pasty, Asda		28	1	80
Chilli Beanfeast, Brooke Bond		28	1	22
Chick Pea Dhal, Sharwood Curry		28	1	40
Chinese Tofu, Granose		28	1	17
Chop Suey: Batchelor's Vesta Meal	portion			478
Chow Mein, Batchelor's Vesta Meal	portion			309

		g	oz	Cal.
Leek & Mushroom Bake, St Michael		28	1	40
Lentil & Bean Bake, Protoveg		28	1	140
Luncheon Roll, Mapletons		28	1	100
Macaroni Cheese, Dalepak	portion			303
Mexican Bean Stew, Granose	tinned	425	15	552
Moussaka, Granose, frozen		28	1	26
Nutbrawn, Granose	tinned	284	10	600
Nut Loaf, Granose	tinned	284	10	500
Potato & Pea Curry, Sharwood		28	1	30
Quorn Chop Suey, Ross		28	1	14
Soya:				
bean curd		28	1	15
bean Frankies, Granose, frozen		28	1	89
bean with onion, Oxo	packet			385
mince with vegetable, Direct Foods, Protoveg Menu		28	1	100
Vegebanger Mix, Realeat, made up	packet			293
Vegeburger Mix, Realeat, made up	packet			240
Vegelinks, Granose		425	15	710

VEGETARIAN DISHES

	g	oz	Cal.
Vegetable Cannelloni, St Michael	28	1	29
Vegetable Curry:			
Mr Fritzi's Frys	28	1	103
Vesta 2 portions			200
Vegetable Goulash, Mr Fritzi's Frys	28	1	103
Vegetable Lasagne, Prewetts	28	1	27
Vegetable Stroganoff, Waitrose	28	1	35

DRINK

	ml	fl oz	Cal.

BEER AND LAGER

	ml	fl oz	Cal.
Arctic Lite Lager, Allied Breweries	284	½pt	82
Carling Black Label, Bass Charrington	568	1pt	220
Carlsberg de Luxe, Carlsberg	275	9¾	122
Carlsberg Special Brew, Carlsberg	284	½pt	205
Carlsen Lite, Carlsberg	275	9¾	85
Colt 45, Courage	440	15½	220
Country Strong Bitter, Ruddles	568	1pt	245
Draught ale: bitter	568	1pt	180
mild	568	1pt	140
Draught Stout, Guinness	568	1pt	182
Export Lager, Watney's	284	½pt	96
Export Ale, Whitbread	454	16	162
Extra Stout, Guinness	284	½pt	110
Forest Brown Ale, Whitbread	440	15½	116
Gerstel Low Alcohol Ale, Courage	330	11½	69
Heineken Lager, Whitbread	275	9¾	77

		ml	fl oz	Cal.
Heldenbrau Lager, Whitbread		275	9¾	61
Hemeling Lager, Bass Charrington		284	½pt	78
Hof Lager, Carlsberg		275	9¾	110
Hofmeister Lager, Courage		275	9¾	96
Ind Coope Double Diamond, Allied Breweries		284	½pt	115
Ind Coope Longlife		284	½pt	101
John Courage	bottle	275	9¾	110
Kaliber		330	11½	59
Kronenbourg Lager: Courage		275	9¾	110
Guinness		284	½pt	110
Harp		568	1pt	255
Limeade & Lager, Corona	can	330	11½	102
Lite Ale, Whitbread		440	15½	76
London Pride, Fullers Beers		284	½pt	105
Mackeson Stout, Whitbread		440	15½	158
McEwan's Export, Scottish & Newcastle		440	15½	150
McEwan's Pale Ale, Scottish & Newcastle		440	15½	103

		ml	fl oz	Cal.
McEwan's Lager, Scottish & Newcastle		440	15½	132
Newcastle Amber Ale, Scottish & Newcastle		275	9¾	70
Newcastle Brown Ale, Scottish & Newcastle		440	15½	170
Pilsner, Carlsberg Lager		284	½pt	75
Red & Special Beer, Watney's	can	440	15½	70
Satzenbrau, Lager: Guinness		284	½pt	106
Harp		275	9¾	110
Shandy: Barr		250	8¾	64
Britvic Slimsta Range		275	9¾	14
Corona	can	140	¼pt	35
'68 Carlsberg Lager		330	11½	200
Skol Lager, Allied Breweries	draught	284	½pt	92
	can	275	9¾	75
Stella Artois, Whitbread Lager	can	330	11½	136
Stones Bitter, Bass Charrington	can	545	16	172
Tankard, Whitbread		284	½pt	100
Tartan Bitter, Scottish & Newcastle	can	440	15½	138
Tartan Special, Scottish & Newcastle	can	440	15½	138

		ml	fl oz	Cal.
Tennent's, Bass Lager	draught	284	½pt	92
Tennent's Extra, Bass Lager	can	440	16	175
Toby Brown Ale, Bass Charrington	bottle	275	9¾	70
Toby Light Ale, Bass Charrington	bottle	275	9¾	70
Worthington E Beer, Bass Charrington		284	½pt	100
Worthington White Shield Beer, Bass Charrington		275	9¾	130
Younger's Lite Ale, Scottish & Newcastle	can	440	15½	106
Younger's Sweet Stout, Scottish & Newcastle	bottle	275	9¾	65

CIDER

	ml	fl oz	Cal.
Autumn Gold Cider, Taunton	284	½pt	118
Dry Blackthorn Cider, Taunton	284	½pt	96
Exhibition Dry Cider, Taunton	284	½pt	150
Exhibition Sweet Cider, Taunton	284	½pt	169

	ml	fl oz	Cal.
Farmhouse Cider, Coates	284	½pt	151
Festival Vat Cider, Coates	284	½pt	135
Norfolk Cider, Gayner's	284	½pt	105
Olde English Cider, Gayner's	284	½pt	124
Pomagne:			
Bulmer's Dry Cider	284	½pt	150
Bulmer's Sweet Cider	284	½pt	184
Pommetta:			
Gayner's Dry Cider	284	½pt	152
Gayner's Sweet Cider	284	½pt	194
Pommia:			
Taunton Dry Cider	284	½pt	156
Taunton Sweet Cider	284	½pt	192
Scrumpy, Coates Cider	284	½pt	126
Somerset, Coates Cider	284	½pt	90
Special Vat, Taunton Cider	284	½pt	121
Strongbow, Bulmer's Cider	284	½pt	101
Strong Dry Cider, Waitrose	284	½pt	94
Woodpecker Cider, Bulmer's	284	½pt	100

		ml	fl oz	Cal.

CRUSHES

		ml	fl oz	Cal.
Bitter Lemon Crush:				
Britvic	bottle	113	4	50
Britvic Slimsta Range	bottle	180	6	0
Blackcurrant Crush, Britvic				
Slimsta Range	bottle	180	6	5
Cariba, Schweppes		330	11½	115
Grapefruit Crush, Britvic				
Slimsta Range	bottle	180	6	11
Lime & Lemon Crush, Britvic	bottle	180	6	85
Orange Crush:				
Britvic	bottle	180	6	84
Britvic Slimsta Range	bottle	180	6	12
Pineapple Crush, Britvic				
Slimsta Range	bottle	180	6	8
Sparkling Orange Crush,				
Schweppes		250	8¾	115

HOT DRINKS

				Cal.
Bournvita, Cadbury	1 teaspoon			22

	ml	fl oz	Cal.
Bovril: 1 teaspoon			12
cube			10
Maxpax Vending Machine	each		15
Build Up, Carnation	sachet	38	1½	135
Chocolate Drink, Maxpax	each			66
Chocolate Flavoured Drink, Drinkmaster	each			70
Chocolate Flavoured Ovaltine	1 teaspoon			16
Cocoa without sugar	1 teaspoon			20
Cocoa powder, average		28	1	15
Coffee & Chicory Essence, Camp	1 teaspoon			10
Coffee beans, average, ground & infused		28g	1oz	0
Coffee: instant, average powder or granules, without water		28	1	28
Maxpax: black with sugar	each			24
with milk, no sugar	each			15
Dandelion Coffee, Lane's Health Products		100g	3½oz	320
Drinking chocolate: average	1 teaspoon			28
Cadbury	1 teaspoon			22
Nisa	1 teaspoon			20

		ml	fl oz	Cal.
Elevenses, Nestlé	1 heaped teaspoon			5
Horlicks Chocolate Malted Low Fat Drink, Beecham	sachet	32g	1½oz	125
Horlicks Malted Drink, Beecham		25	1	96
Hot Chocolate, Wimpy	each			230
Hot Chocolate Mix, Carnation		29g	1oz	110
Lemon Tea:				
Drinkmaster Vending Machine	each			40
Maxpax	each			35
Low Fat Drinking Chocolate Granules, St Michael		28g	1oz	102
Malted Chocolate Flavour Drink, Batchelor's Cup-a-Time	sachet			125
Malted Drink, Boots	per cup			119
Malted Milk, Safeway	1 teaspoon			35
Malt Flavour Drink, Batchelor's Cup-a-Time	sachet			132
Marvel, Cadbury, dry	1 teaspoon			6
Milk:				
fresh, pasteurized, Silver Top		568	1pt	380

	ml	fl oz	Cal.
instant, Tesco: dry		28g	1oz	103
made up		575	1pt	192
Milquick, St Ivel	1 teaspoon			6
Nesquik, Nestlé		28g	1oz	108
Ovaltine, Wander: granules	1 teaspoon			20
powder	sachet	20g	¾oz	80
Oxo Beef Drink, Brooke Bond Oxo	1 teaspoon			4
cube				16
Oxo Chicken Cube, Brooke Bond Oxo	cube			16
Slim Choc, Carnation	sachet			41
Tea, Drinkmaster Vending Machine: white with sugar	each			40
white, no sugar	each			10
Tea-Mate, Carnation	1 teaspoon			10
White Freeze-dried Coffee, Maxpax	each			21
White Tea, no sugar, Maxpax	each			9

		ml	fl oz	Cal.

JUICES

Apple Juice:

Copella	carton	200	7	86
Del Monte	carton	142	¼pt	61
Gateway		100	3½	38
Southern Gold Long Life		140	¼pt	64

Apple & Honey Drink, Hi-Fruit Still Fruit Drinks		28	1	14
Barley Cup, Ridpath Pek	1 teaspoon			6
Beetroot Juice, Biotta	1 litre			400
Carrot Juice, Biotta		100	4	35
Coconut milk, fresh		28	1	6
Five Alive Citrus Juice, Coca Cola		200	7	95
Five Alive Tropical, Coca Cola		200	7	85
Florida Orange Juice, Birds Eye reconstituted		140	¼pt	43
Good Start Juice, Libby's		140	¼pt	51

Grapefruit Juice:

Britvic	bottle	113	4	62
Britvic '55'	bottle	180	6	90
Club	bottle	113	4	65
Express Dairies		140	¼pt	43

		ml	fl oz	Cal.
Just Juice		140	¼pt	50
Southern Gold, Longlife		140	¼pt	55
Grape Juice: Bulmer's		140	¼pt	66
Schloer		250	8¾	123
Hi-C Orange Juice, Coca Cola		200	7	91
Jaffa Orange Juice, St Michael		200	7	60
Natural Apple Juice, Martlett		100	4	40
Orange Juice:				
average, unsweetened		28	1	11
Britvic		113	4	49
Club, sweetened	bottle	113	4	61
Club, unsweetened	bottle	113	4	57
Express Dairies		100	4	35
Heinz		120	4¼	56
Libby's unsweetened		140	¼pt	45
Robinson's, Ready Drink		250	8¾	92
Waitrose		200	7	84
Zing		180	6¼	89
Orange, Apple & Passion Fruit, Del Monte		140	¼pt	59
Pineapple Juice:				
Britvic '55'	can	250	8¾	127
Canada Dry, Sodastream	bottle	113	4	55
Club	bottle	113	4	62
Del Monte		100	3.5	46
Sainsbury		140	¼pt	62

DRINK

		ml	fl oz	Cal.
Prune juice, average		28	1	26
Red Grape Juice, Schloer	carton	250	8¾	123
Sun & Rise Juice, Kellogg's:				
lemon, reconstituted		113	4	45
orange, pineapple,				
blackcurrant, reconstituted		113	4	50
Sunfruit Juice, St Michael		140	¼pt	68
Tomato Juice: average		28	1	6
Club	bottle	113	4	25
Libby		115	4.2	19
Unsweetened Orange, Club	bottle	113	4	48

MILK SHAKES

		ml	fl oz	Cal.
Banana Milk Shake, Crusha		28	1	30
Chocolate Shake, McDonald's	each			303
Strawberry Milk, St Michael		150	6½	140
Strawberry Shake, McDonald's	each			312
Thick Shake, Wimpy	each			250
Two Shakes Chocolate Drink Mix, Kellogg's	sachet			75

		ml	fl oz	Cal.
Vanilla Shake, McDonald's	each			301
Whippsy, Wimpy	each			222

NON-ALCOHOLIC DRINKS

		ml	fl oz	Cal.
Apple & Blackcurrant Drink, Robinson		250	8¾	112
Applesparkle, St Michael	can	100		47
Appletise, Schweppes	bottle	180	7	75
Beer Shandy, non-alcoholic, Minster	can	270	9½	70
Bitter Lemon: Canada Dry	bottle	175	6	70
Club	bottle	113	4	30
	bottle	180	7	50
Hunts, sparkling		140	¼pt	50
Sainsbury		140	¼pt	45
Spar		100	4	43
Waitrose		100	4	35
Cherryade, Whites		28	1	6
Cherry Coca Cola	can	330	11½	140
Coca Cola, Coca Cola		330	11½	130

		ml	fl oz	Cal.
Coke: Pizza Express	each			110
Wimpy	large			133
Cola: Britvic		110	4	43
Canada Dry	bottle			60
Sainsbury		280	½pt	120
Cream Soda, Whites		28	1	5
Danish Life, non-alcoholic lager		320	1	57
Diet Coca Cola, Coca Cola		330	11½	0
Diet Pepsi, Pepsi Cola		330	11½	0
Dry Ginger Ale: average		100	4	14
Safeway		140	¼pt	34
Waitrose		140	¼pt	30
Duo Club		180	6	72
Fanta Cream Soda, Coca Cola	1 litre		1¾pt	292
Fanta Ginger Beer, Coca Cola	1 litre		1¾pt	310
Fanta Lemonade, Coca Cola	can	330	11½	80
Fanta Limeade, Coca Cola	1 litre		1¾pt	240
Fanta Orangeade, Coca Cola		330	11½	112
Fanta Raspberryade, Coca Cola	1 litre		1¾pt	296
Ginger Beer: average		28	1	11
Corona	bottle	140	¼pt	40
Schweppes	bottle	170	5½	60

NON-ALCOHOLIC DRINKS

		ml	fl oz	Cal.
Hi-Juice 66, Schweppes		250	8½	130
Indian Tonic Water: Hunts		140	¼pt	34
Idris		140	¼pt	34
Irn Bru, Barr		250	8¾	100
Jusoda Orange Drink, Barr	bottle	250	8¾	89
Lemonade:				
Barr		250	8¾	65
Boots Shapers	can	330	11½	0
Britvic	bottle	113	4	34
Britvic Slimsta Range	bottle	170	6	5
Canada Dry Slim Drink		175	6¼	0
Corona		100	3½	39
Whites		100	3½	20
Lemonade Shandy, Schweppes		275	½pt	68
Lemon Drink, Drinkmaster Vending Machine	each			58
Lemon Countrytime Drink, Maxpax	each			25
Lemon & Limeade, Sodastream, made up		230	8	63
Lemonade Shandy, Safeway	can	330	11½	128
Limeade, Tesco		140	¼pt	52
Lilt, Coca Cola		330	11½	162
Lucozade	bottle	250	8½	180

		ml	fl oz	Cal.
Mineral water, average				0
Orange & Apple Drink, Robinsons		250	8¾	90
Orange & Apricot Drink, Waitrose		140	¼pt	53
Orange Drink, Drinkmaster Vending Machine	each			50
Orange Sixty, Rawlings		180	6	102
Pineapple Sixty, Rawlings	bottle	180	6	102
Pepsi Cola, Pepsi Cola	can	330	11½	145
Raspberry, Zing		180	6¼	80
Russchian, Schweppes	bottle	500	17½	115
Seven up:		341	12	130
diet		341	12	0
Shandy: Barr		250	8¾	64
Britvic Slimsta Range		275	9¾	14
Corona	can	140	¼pt	35
Slimgard Liquid Meal Replacement, strawberry	meal			325
Slimline: American Ginger Ale, Schweppes	bottle	180	6¼	0

		ml	fl oz	Cal.
Bitter Lemon, Schweppes	bottle	180	6¼	4
Lemonade & Beer Shandy, Schweppes	bottle	330	11½	19
Lemonade, Schweppes	bottle	180	6¼	0
Sparkling Orange Crush, Schweppes	bottle	330	11½	6
Tonic Water, Schweppes	bottle	180	6¼	0
Sparkling Bitter Lemon Drink:				
Hunts	bottle	140	¼pt	47
Hunts low calorie	bottle	250	8¾	0
Schweppes	bottle	180	6¼	59
Sparkling Blackcurrantade, Corona	bottle	140	¼pt	36
Sparkling Cherryade, Corona	bottle	250	8¾	63
Sparkling Cola Drink, Corona	bottle	250	8¾	103
Sparkling Cream Soda, Corona	bottle	140	¼pt	36
Sparkling Pineapple & Grapefruit Drink, Tango	can	330	11½	145
Sparkling Iron Brew, Corona		140	¼pt	28
Sparkling Lemon & Lime Drink, Hunts low calorie	can	250	8¾	9
Sparkling Limeade, Corona	can	140	¼pt	32
Sparkling Orangeade, Corona	can	140	¼pt	39

		ml	fl oz	Cal.
Sparkling Orange Drink, Hunts low calorie	can	250	8¾	10
Sparkling Orange & Pineapple Drink, Tango	can	330	11½	146
low calorie		100	4	2
Strawberry Drink, Cresta		250	8¾	90
Strike Cola, Barr	bottle	250	8¾	85
Tab, Coca Cola	can			0
Tango: Orange	can	100	4	45
Lemon with Lime	can	100	4	35
Tizer, Barr	can	250	8¾	100
	can	330	11½	130
Tomato Cocktail, Club	bottle	113	4	25
Tonic Water:				
Canada Dry	bottle	175	6¼	40
Canada Dry Slim Drink	bottle	175	6¼	0
Schweppes Slimline Drink	bottle	180	6¼	0
Wine, de-alcoholized	average glass	115	4	35

		ml	fl oz	Cal.

SLIMMERS' AND HEALTH DRINKS

		ml	fl oz	Cal.
Bitter Lemon:				
Boots low calorie	can	330	11½	5
Hunts low calorie		140	¼pt	5
Bittersweet sparkling low calorie drinks	can	250	8¾	10
Schweppes Slimline	bottle	180	6¼	5
Sainsbury low calorie		100	4	½
Butterscotch Complan	serving	57g	2oz	250
Carob Night Time Drink	powder	30g	1oz	97
Chocolate Complan, Complan		57g	2oz	252
Chocolate Flavour Cup-a-Time, Batchelor's	sachet			120
Cola: Boots low calorie		330	11½	5
Britvic Slimsta Range		180	6	8
Dandelion & Burdock, Whites		28	1	7
Diet Coca Cola, Coca Cola		330	11½	0
Diet Lemonade, Whites		250	8¾	1
Diet Pepsi Cola, Pepsi Cola		330	11½	0
Diet Ginger Ale, Safeway		140	¼pt	6
Grapefruit C, Libby's		140	¼pt	54

DRINK

		ml	fl oz	Cal.
Irn Bru, low calorie, Barr		330	11½	16
Kaltenberg Diet Pils, Whitbread		284	½pt	119
Lemonade:				
Boots Shapers, Cloudy	can	330	11½	1
Canada Dry Slim Drink		175	6	0
Lemon & Lime, Boots low calorie drink	can	330	11½	5
Lemon Squash, Roses, diabetic		28	1	0
Low Calorie:				
American Ginger Ale, Hunts		140	¼pt	0
Bitter Lemon, Hunts		140	¼pt	0
Bitter Orange, Hunts		142	¼pt	4
Indian Tonic Water		140	¼pt	0
Jaffa Lemon Drink, Tesco		28	1	5
Orange Crush, St Michael		250	8¾	9
Tonic, Club		113	4	0
Tonic Water, Sainsbury		100	3½	½
Pils, Holstein Diabetic Lager		270	9	106
Plamil C Soya Milk Concentrate		30	1	29
Pranavite Slim, HTB (UK) Milk Protein drink	sachet			200
Seven Up, diet		341	12	0
Slim Choc, Carnation	sachet			41

		ml	fl oz	Cal.
Slimline:				
American Ginger Ale, Schweppes	bottle	180	6¼	0
Bitter Lemon, Schweppes	bottle	180	6¼	4
Lemonade & Beer Shandy, Schweppes	bottle	330	11½	19
Lemonade, Schweppes	bottle	180	6¼	0
Sparkling Orange Crush, Schweppes	bottle	330	11¼	6
Tonic Water, Schweppes	bottle	180	6¼	0
Soya Milk, Granose		140	¼pt	74
Sparkling Bitter Lemon Drink, Hunts low calorie	bottle	250	8¾	0
Sparkling Dandelion & Burdock, Corona	bottle	140	¼pt	28
Sparkling Lemon & Lime Drink, Hunts low calorie	can	250	8¾	9
Sparkling Orange Drink, Hunts low calorie	can	250	8¾	10
Strawberry Milk Drink, low fat, Unigate		568	1pt	335
Tonic Water:				
Canada Dry Slim Drink	bottle	175	6¼	0
Schweppes Slimline Drink	bottle	180	6¼	0

	ml	fl oz	Cal.

SPIRITS, LIQUEURS AND FORTIFIED WINES

	ml	fl oz	Cal.
Advocaat	25	⅙ gill	65
Apricot brandy	25	⅙ gill	60
Brandy	25	⅙ gill	50
Calvados	25	⅙ gill	65
Campari	25	⅙ gill	57
Champagne: average	110	4	80
Safeway	110	4	105
Chartreuse	25	⅙ gill	100
Cherry brandy	25	⅙ gill	64
Cinzano: Bianco	50	⅓ gill	82
Rosso	50	⅓ gill	76
Cointreau	25	⅙ gill	85
Cream sherry	50	⅓ gill	65
Crème de cassis	25	⅙ gill	60
Crème de menthe	35	⅙ gill	82
Crocodillo	bottle		61
Curaçao	25	⅙ gill	70

	ml	fl oz	Cal.
Drambuie	25	⅙ gill	80
Dry sherry	50	⅓ gill	59
Dubonnet: dry	50	⅓ gill	55
red	50	⅓ gill	70
Frattelli Bianco, Vermouth	50	⅓ gill	74
Galliano	25	⅙ gill	76
Gin	25	⅙ gill	55
Ginger wine	113	4	185
Goldwell's Calypso, low alcohol drink	bottle		102
Goldwell's Wee McGlen, low alcohol drink	bottle		102
Grand Marnier	25	⅙ gill	80
Kirsch	25	⅙ gill	47
Kümmel	25	⅙ gill	75
Malibu	25	⅙ gill	51
Margarita, Shakers	bottle 160	6½	160
Martini Bianco	50	⅓ gill	67
Martini Extra Dry	50	⅓ gill	67
Martini Rosé	50	⅓ gill	85

DRINK

	ml	fl oz	Cal.
Martini Rosso	50	⅓ gill	91
Pernod	25	⅙ gill	61
Pimms No I Cup	50	⅓ gill	98
Pina Colada, St Michael	250	8¾	230
Port	25	⅙ gill	36
Rum	25	⅙ gill	55
Sherry: cream	50	⅓ gill	63
dry	50	⅓ gill	54
medium	50	⅓ gill	58
Strega	25	⅙ gill	77
Tequila	25	⅙ gill	50
Tia Maria	25	⅙ gill	75
Vodka	25	⅙ gill	53
Whisky	25	⅙ gill	50

SQUASHES

	ml	fl oz	Cal.
Barley Water, Robinson's, undiluted	28	I	30
Beetroot squash	100	3½	40

SQUASHES

		ml	fl oz	Cal.
Blackcurrant: Cresta		28	1	10
	1 litre		1¾pt	50
	bottle	250	8¾	90
Drinkmaster Vending Machine	each			30
Maxpax	each			25
Blackcurrant Drink:				
Waitrose, undiluted		28	1	65
C Vit, undiluted		28	1	42
Ribena, undiluted		28	1	80
Caribbean Fruit Drink, Hi-Fruit Still Fruit Drink		28	1	14
Lemon Barley Water, Tesco, undiluted		100		107
Lemon Squash, undiluted:				
average		28	1	30
Roses Diabetic		28	1	1.5
Ribena, Beecham:				
Baby, all flavours		28	1	90
concentrated ready to drink		28	1	80
Whole grapefruit drink, diluted with water, average		28	1	30
Whole lemon drink, diluted with water, average		28	1	26

	ml	fl oz	Cal.
Whole orange drink, diluted with water, average	28	1	32

SYRUPS AND CORDIALS

	ml	fl oz	Cal.
Banana Syrup, Rayner/Burgess	28	1	61
Blackcurrant Cordial, Corona, undiluted	100	3½	100
Blackcurrant Flavour Cordial, Corona, undiluted	28	1	60
Chocolate Milk Shake Syrup, Crusha	28	1	47
Ginger cordial, undiluted	28	1	27
Grenadine syrup	28	1	72
Pineapple milk shake syrup	1 tablespoon		20
Raspberry Milk Shake Syrup, Crusha	28	1	30
Rosehip syrup, undiluted	100	3½	232
	1 tablespoon		95
Red Grape Juice, sparkling, Schloer	225	7½	110
Strawberry cordial, undiluted	28	1	34